The ABC of Traditional Chinese Medicine

By Shi Jizong & Chu Feng Zhu
Translated by Shi Jiaxin

HAI FENG PUBLISHING COMPANY
HONGKONG

© **Hai Feng Publishing Co. 1985**
ISBN 962-238-036-0

Published by
Hai Feng Publishing Co.
17/F., Paramount Building,
12 Kai Yip Street, Chai Wan,
Hong Kong

Printed by
Friendly Printing Co., Ltd.
Flat B1, 3/F., Luen Ming Hing Ind. Bldg.,
36 Muk Cheong St., Tokwawan, Kowloon,
Hong Kong

Fourth Edition 1992

HF-54-P

Contents

Chapter 1	**Chinese Medicine — A Medicine of Long-Standing**	1
Chapter 2	**Physiology and Pathology**	6
2.1	*Qi*, blood, body fluid	6
2.2	Channels and collaterals	8
2.3	Viscera and bowels	10
Chapter 3	**Methods of Diagnosis**	11
3.1	Inspection	11
3.2	Ausculation	14
3.3	Interrogation	15
3.4	Palpation	20
Chapter 4	**Causes of Diseases**	28
4.1	Wind and cold	28
4.2	Summer heat and dampness	29
4.3	Dryness and fire	29
4.4	Internal injury	30
Chapter 5	**Principles of Treatment and Differentiation of Symptom-Complexes**	31
5.1	Incidental or fundamental, greater or lesser urgent cases	31
5.2	Adjusting *yin* and *yang*	32
5.3	Difference of symptoms and their transformation	33

5.4 Consideration of medical treatment based on various conditions	34
Chapter 6 Eight Methods of Treatment	37
6.1 Diaphoretic method	37
6.2 Emetic method	39
6.3 Purgation method	39
6.4 Mediation method	40
6.5 Febrifugal method	41
6.6 Warming method	41
6.7 Elimination method	42
6.8 Tonifying method	42
Chapter 7 Eight Principal Syndromes	44
7.1 Exterior and interior	45
7.2 Cold and heat	46
7.3 Deficiency and excessiveness	47
7.4 *Yin* and *yang*	48
Chapter 8 Seven Prescriptions	49
8.1 Heavy and mild prescriptions	50
8.2 Slow-acting and quick-acting prescriptions	50
8.3 Prescriptions with one principal ingredient and those with two or more principal ingredients	51
8.4 Compound prescriptions	52
Chapter 9 Chinese Traditional Drugs	53
9.1 Four properties of drugs	53
9.2 Five tastes of drugs	54
9.3 Combination of drugs	55
9.4 Contraindications	56
Chapter 10 Common Diseases and Their Prevention and Cure	59
10.1 Treatment of influenza	59

10.2	Treatment of stomach trouble	64
10.3	Treatment of nausea and vomiting during early pregnancy	65
10.4	Treatment of tracheitis caused by cold	66
10.5	Recipe for chronic bronchitis	67
10.6	Recipe for threatened abortion	67
10.7	Recipe for bed-wetting	68
10.8	Recipe for infant constipation	68
10.9	Recipe for insomnia	68
10.10	Recipe for contraception	68
10.11	Recipe for old people's constipation	69
10.12	Treatment of coronary heart disease	69
10.13	Tonics for old people	69
10.14	Blood tonics	70
10.15	Ten recipes of Dr. Shi Jinmo	71
	10.15.1 *Recipe for cirrhosis of the liver*	71
	10.15.2 *Recipe for oedematous liver or spleen*	71
	10.15.3 *Recipe for gastric ulcer*	72
	10.15.4 *Recipe for duodenal ulcer*	72
	10.15.5 *Recipe for chronic dysentery*	72
	10.15.6 *Recipe for chronic enteritis*	73
	10.15.7 *Recipe for cirrhosis with ascites*	73
	10.15.8 *Recipe for cirrhosis with jaundice*	73
	10.15.9 *Recipe for cholelith and jaundice*	74
	10.15.10 *Recipe for dilatation and ptosis of the stomach*	74

Chapter 11 Records of Shi Jinmo's Clinical Practice — 76

11.1	Treatment of stomach trouble	77
11.2	Treatment of hypertension	81
11.3	Treatment of neurasthenia	83
11.4	Treatment of migraine	85
11.5	Treatment of diabetes: dietetic and medical	87
11.6	Treatment of urological diseases	91
11.7	Treatment of impotence	98
11.8	Treatment of diarrhea of old people	100
11.9	Treatment of otitis media	102

11.10	Treatment of gout	104
11.11	Treatment of dysmenorrhoea	107
11.12	Treatment of tubercular erythema	109
11.13	Treatment of purpura	111
11.14	Treatment of typhus	115
Appendix:	**English and/or Latin Names of Chinese Drugs in Common Use**	117

Foreword

Traditional Chinese medicine has a very long history and that makes it difficult for the people of today. This book intends to explain its history, its characteristics and clinical practice in plain language. The book also introduces the principles of treatment and methods of diagnosis of traditional Chinese medical science, annotates different properties, effects, etc. of traditional Chinese drugs, together with eight methods of treatment. A number of patent medicines and commonly used recipes are also recommended.

Included in the book is an introduction to Shi Jinmo, a famous doctor of traditional Chinese medicine of the present time, and some of his prescriptions.

Translating the names of Chinese drugs, about 300 of them in this book, has been a difficult job. The translator's concern is that the reader who does not know Chinese should be enabled to know what they are in Latin or English and to get them in Chinese pharmacies. So the drugs' names are given in Chinese phonetic alphabet in the text of the book, while the Index offers their Latin and English equivalents. For those without proper equivalents, necessary explanations are given to make them comprehensible.

Except notified otherwise, the prescriptions or recipes introduced in the book refer to decoctions of medicinal ingredients, i.e. medicine prepared by boiling to be taken after the drugs are removed.

Chapter 1

Chinese Medicine — A Medicine of Long-Standing

Traditional Chinese medicine has a long history. Internal diseases were recorded by the most ancient language — inscriptions on the bones or tortoise shells of the Shang Dynasty (c. 16th − 11th century B.C.) Diseases involving the heart, head, intestines and stomach as well as epidemic diseases, for instance, were mentioned in the oracle-bone inscriptions. In fact, in the latter period of the Shang Dynasty, medicine prepared by boiling was used in treating internal diseases. The word "medical master" which referred to physicians first appeared in the *Zhou Book of Rites* 周禮, a book published in the Zhou Dynasty (c. 11th century − 256 B.C.). By then, Chinese medical men had found seasonal diseases such as excessive dandruff in spring, scabies in summer, malaria in autumn and coughing in winter. Pestilence was also found about the same time.

All these show that China's medical science had already developed considerably as early as the Zhou Dynasty, when internal medicine had become an independent branch. Seasonal diseases were treated and drugs were used. The traditional four methods of diagnosis, namely, inspection (望, Wang), auscultation (聞, Wen), interrogation (問, Wen), and pulse feeling (切, Qie), came into being also at that time.

The oldest medical classic of China is called *Huangdi Neijing* ("Huangdi's Internal Classic", or "Canon of Medicine" 《黄帝内經》). With its authorship ascribed to the ancient emperor *Huangdi* (2698 – 2589 B.C.), the work was a product of various unknown authors in the Warring States Period (475 – 221 B.C.). Consisting of two parts – "Plain Questions" 《素問》 and "Miraculous Pivot" 靈樞 – it recorded diseases of respirators and of digestive, urinary and reproductive organs as well as epidemic diseases. It also put forward the theory of metabolism. In treating internal diseases, the book offered methods of using drugs opposite in nature to the symptom-complex or of the same nature as that of the pseudo-symptom-complex. Although it contains only 13 prescriptions, the book is still prized by physicians of today because of its variety of subjects.

Ancient China produced numerous distinguished physicians. One of the earliest was Bian Que 扁鵲 (about 500 B.C.), who was good at various subjects, especially in internal diseases. Once he saved a prince from "shijue" 尸厥, an ancient term for shock. He was also an initiator of pulse-taking. *Difficult Classic* 《難經》, a book on 81 difficult problems of medicine, is said to be written by Bian Que.

Hua Tuo 華陀 (? – 208 A.D.) of the Han Dynasty was the most famous surgeon and also master of internal medicine, surgery, gynaecology, paediatrics, acupuncture, etc. – almost every branch of medicine. Called by the people "miracle-working doctor", he was said to have performed many major operations including abdominal section with herbal anesthesia. He also attached importance to taking exercise and recommended therapeutic gymnastics called the Frolics of Five Animals. He held that the smooth circulation of blood was imperative for health.

Among other distinguished physicians was Zhang Zhongjing 張仲景 (also called Zhang Ji, 150 – 219 A.D.) of the Han Dynasty, who wrote *Treatiese on Febrile and Miscellaneous Diseases* and *Synopsis of Prescriptions of the*

Golden Chamber 《金匱要略》. He has been considered the founder of the principle of treating diseases according to the method of differentiating symptoms and signs.

Wang Shuhe 王叔和 (about 210 − 285 A.D.) of the Jin Dynasty rearranged Zhang Zhongjing's *Treatise on Febrile and Miscellaneous Diseases* into ten volumes, differentiated febrile diseases from miscellaneous diseases, and wrote that as a separate section *Treatise on Febrile Diseases*. In that book he perfected and systematized Zhang's theory and divided the diseases into six stages, and offered 397 methods and 113 recipes in treating them. He confirmed the Eight Principle Syndromes, i.e. *Yin* and *Yang*, exterior and interior, heat and cold, insufficiency and excessiveness. (See Chapter 5) Wang Shuhe 王叔和 wrote *The Pulse Classic* 《脈經》, which is considered the first comprehensive book on sphygmology now extant in China.

Most famous of the Sui Dynasty was Chao Yuanfang 巢元方, an imperial physician who took charge of the compilation of the well-known 50-volume *General Treatise on the Etiology Symptomatology of Diseases* 《諸病源候論》, in 610 A.D.; which was the first Chinese work in this category and is still much valued.

The Peaceful Holy Benevolent Prescriptions 《太平聖惠方》 and the *Imperial Encyclopaedia of Medicine* 《聖濟總錄》 are works of the Northern Song Dynasty (960 − 1127 A.D.). The former, compiled by Wang Huaiyin 王懷隱, included 16,834 prescriptions of various medical branches with discussions on diagnosis and pathology of different diseases.

In the Southern Song Dynasty (1127 − 1279), Chen Yan 陳言 (also called Chen Wuze) advanced the three categories of pathology: endogenous, exogenous and non-exo-endogenous. The endogenous causes of disease referred chiefly to the excessive emotional changes − joy, anger, melancholy, anxiety, sorrow, fear and fright. Exogenous causes referred to the six excessive and untimely atmospheric influences: wind, cold, summer heat, dampness, dryness and fire. Non-exo-endogenous causes meant those related neither to external nor to internal influences, such as intemperance in eating, drinking and sexual life, overwork, animal bite, etc. Chen's theory promoted ancient China's research on etiology. Chen was the author of the book *A Treatise on the Three Categories of Pathogenic Factors of Diseases* 《三因極一病症方論》, a work of 18 volumes published in 1174.

The Ming (1368 – 1644) and Qing (1644 – 1911) Dynasties saw a big development in medical science. The greatest work at this time was the 168-volume *Prescriptions for Universal Relief* 《普濟方》, an encyclopaedia of internal medicine with 61,739 prescriptions and 239 illustrations. It was written by Teng Hong et al. under the patronage of Zhu Su 朱橚 and was issued in 1406 A.D.

In the Qing Dynasty, theories on acute febrile diseases further developed.

During the Taiping Heavenly Kingdom (1851 – 1864), the noted doctor Wu Shangxian 吳尚先 (1806 – 1866) initiated economical methods of treatment for those in the countryside who could not afford high charges for medical care and advocated external therapies, such as ointment and plasters, hydrotherapy, breathing therapy, cautery and moxibustion. He was the author of *A Rhymed Discourse on New Therapeutics* 《外治醫說》 (1864 A.D.).

China's minority nationalities also developed their traditional medicine long ago. The Uygurs, for instance, used plants, minerals, animal meat and bones and cheese in treating diseases, as early as the second and third centuries. Before the Han Dynasty, their caravans were already equipped with professional doctors. Among a few medical works left behind are two books on examination of both living and dead human bodies, written by Pasilaha in the eighth century. After more than 2,000 years of practice, Uygur medicine had developed into a complete theoretical system based on a unique environment. They used fire, air, water and earth to stand for materials, and believed that four different fluids (blood, phlegm, bile and black fluid) existed in the human body, and they based their theory on such understanding.

The theory and practice of Chinese traditional medicine, which has been recorded by numerous works over the past several thousand years, is an important component of China's national culture. This book, the purpose of which is to help readers gain a rough idea about traditional Chinese medicine, will go on to explain its theory, causes of disease, differentiation of symptom-complexes, methods of treatment and prescriptions.

Chapter 2
Physiology and Pathology

Based on the anatomy of ancient people, Chinese traditional medicine has two hypotheses about physiology and pathology:

First, the human body is composed of viscera and bowels, channels and collaterals, *Qi* (vital energy 氣), blood, body fluid, skin and hairs, blood vessels, tendons and bones, as well as the five sense organs (ears, eyes, lips, nose and tongue) and orifices (or openings) at the front and back private parts.

Secondly, the five viscera (heart, liver, spleen, lung and kidney) and the six bowels (gallbladder, stomach, large intestine, small intestine, urinary bladder and the Triple Burners*) are connected with and restrict each other, through the main and collateral channels and the vital energy and blood flowing in them.

The theory consists of the following three parts.

2.1 *QI*, BLOOD, BODY FLUID

---

* The Triple Burners (or Heaters, 三焦) refer to the three portions of the body cavity. The Upper Burner: the upper portion of the body cavity, the part above the diaphragm of the body cavity housing the heart and the lung; the Middle Burner: the portion between the diaphragm and umbilicus of the body cavity housing the spleen and the stomach; the Lower Burner: the portion below umbilicus of the body cavity housing the kidney, urinary bladder, small and large intestines, etc.

The concept of *Qi* represents the elementary understanding of natural phenomena in ancient times. In the field of medicine, *Qi* is referred to as the basic element or energy which makes up the human body and supports vital activities, such as food energy, inspired air, the functional activities of viscera and bowels, and the vital function of the channels of the body.

Qi (vital energy) and blood have different functions but are related to each other. Vital energy is believed to be the "commander" of blood: it serves as the dynamic force of blood flow. Blood is the "mother" of the vital energy by being the latter's material basis.

Vital energy has many forms of expression, the most important of which is "original vital energy" 元氣, as the motive force of all visceral functions. The original vital energy consists of air which the human body absorbs through the lung, and food energy transformed through the spleen and stomach. In that sense, the vital energy is a kind of material which can move to every part of the human body.

Inside the human body, there is also a "defensive energy" 衛氣, which moves outside the conduits, permeating the surface of the body and warding off exogenous pathogens.

Doctors observe illness according to the physiological action of the vital energy. Weak breathing, for instance, indicates deficiency of vital energy of the lung and having no appetite means deficiency of vital energy of the stomach and spleen. The imbalance of vital energy in upward and downward movements gives rise to illness.

Blood is derived by transformation of the food essence which is transformed through the heart and lung. A medical classic describes blood as "the red fluid originating from the Middle Burner after transformation." Here, the Middle Burner refers to the spleen and stomach and "transformation" means the function of the heart and lung.

Pathologically, there are deficiency of blood, stasis of blood, and stagnant heat in the blood system. Deficiency of blood is caused by the decrease of blood sources or the excessive loss of blood. Impeded circulation, injuries, deficiency of vital energy as well as stagnant heat and invasion of cold into the blood may lead to the stasis of blood. Stagnant heat in the blood system, caused by the invasion of blood by noxious heat, leads to macula on the human body or even unconsciousness.

Body fluid plays an important role in the human body. It is distributed all over the body and is important in moistening internal organs, skin and muscle, lubricating joints and nourishing the brains. Impairment of body fluid means lack of fluid. The symptoms are thirst, dry cough irritability, scanty urine, constipation, etc.

2.2 CHANNELS AND COLLATERALS

There exists within the human body a system of channels through which the vital energy and blood circulate, and by which the internal organs are connected with superficial organs and tissues, as well as the right with the left and upper with below. The body is thus made an organic whole.

Channels (meridians 經) are cardinal conduits of vital energy and blood coursing vertically. Collaterals (reticular conduits 絡) are the branches of the channels. The whole system consists of Twelve Channels*, and Eight Extra Channels**, collaterals or branches of the Twelve Regular Channels***, Fifteen Main Collaterals of the Channels****, tertiary collaterals muscles distributed along the Twelve Regular Channels and the Skin Zones or cutaneous regions of the Twelve Regular Channels.*****

Abnormal function of the channels can spread illness to a certain part of the body. Cold in the exterior, for instance, can affect the lung and cause cough, phlegm and pain in the chest. Similarly, kidney trouble may affect the waist, and liver disease may give rise to pain in the costal region.

The theory of channels is widely used in clinical practice. It is the basis of acupuncture and moxibustion. When someone is ill, the physician can regulate the flow of vital energy and blood by puncturing, massaging or applying medicine to certain points on his body surface and thus cure the illness of the associated internal organs.

Acupuncture anaesthesia can relieve pain and can also prevent it. Acupuncture, moxibustion and massage often can cure diseases before which medicine is helpless.

---

* The Twelve Channels 十二經絡 , known as the Regular Channels, each being connected with a particular internal organ and each possessing an exterior-interior relation, are:
  the Lung Channel of Hand *Taiyin* 太陰; the Large Intestine Channel of Hand *Yangming* 陽明; the Stomach Channel of Foot *Yangming*; the Spleen Channel of Foot *Taiyin*; the Heart Channel of Hand *Shaoying* 少陰; etc.

** The Eight Extra Channels 奇經八脈 , also called the Eight Odd Conduits, stand for:

  the Front Middle Channel, the Back Middle Channel, the Vital Channel, the Belt Channel, the Motility Channel of *Yin* 陰, the Motility Channel of *Yang* 陽, the Regulating Channel of *Yin*, and the Regulating Channel of *Yang*.

They are not directly connected with the internal organs. Their physiological function is to help regulate and keep in reserve the vital energy and blood circulating in the Twelve Channels.

*** The collaterals (branches of the Twelve Regular Channels 十二經別 run in the deep part of the body to strengthen the communication between the interior and exterior channels of the Twelve Regular Channels in the trunk, and serve as a supplementary passage for the flow of vital energy of the Regular Channels.

**** The Fifteen Main Collaterals of the Channels 十五絡脈 : each of the Fourteen Channels has a collateral and together with the Great Collateral of the Spleen make up the Fifteen Main Collaterals, which communicate with the exterior and the interior of the body.

***** The Skin Zones (cutaneous regions) of the Twelve Regular Channels 十二經筋 : the Skin Zones reflect the functioning condition of the Channels. Pathologically, pathogenic factors may get into the body from the cutaneous regions to the interior channels. On the contrary, if an internal organ is deseased, it may be made known by changes on the Skin Zone through which the channels and collaterals run.

2.3 VISCERA AND BOWELS

The theory of Viscera and Bowels deals with the physiological functions and pathological changes of the internal organs. The five viscera, namely, heart, liver, spleen, lung and kidney, install essence and energy and maintain the physiological activities of the human body.

The six bowels refer to gallbladder, stomach, large intestine, small intestine, urinary bladder and the triple burners. They are supposed to receive and digest food, supply the viscera with food essence and discharge the waste from the body.

The five viscera and six bowels, plus the pericardium which surrounds the heart, are also called the "Twelve Viscera" (十二藏).

The viscera and bowels are related to each other and condition each other. The function of the heart, for instance, is connected with that of the brain. The heart also has internal connection with the tongue, as one classic put it: "The tongue is the body opening to the heart." The function of tendons and tendon sheaths is believed to be controlled by the liver and has influence on the stomach. Hence differentiation of symptom-complexes.

Chapter 3

Methods of Diagnosis

Inspection (望), auscultation (聞) (or audio-olfactive investigation), interrogation (問) and palpation (切) (or pulse-feeling) are the four basic diagnostic methods of physicians of Chinese medicine in clinical practice. These are ways to judge causes and mechanisms of disease — the internal or external location of the illness; the cold or heat of the pathogenic factors; the deficiency or excessiveness of the symptom-complexes. They are also ways to help decide how to treat diseases and anticipate their result.

3.1 INSPECTION

Inspection is examination by the eye. It is the first step for the physician to judge the patient's general condition in diagnosis. The first impression can be obtained from inspecting the patient's complexion, and facial expression. The inspection may also include lustre of the eye, behaviour, skin, eyes, ears, tongue, throat, and even the patient's phlegm, stool, urine, etc.

This will be elaborated in the following.

3.1.1 Inspection of complexion and facial expressions

The change of skin colour, or complexion may serve as

outward manifestation of the patient's illness. There are mainly five colours — blue, red, yellow, white and black — that reveal illness in corresponding viscera, i.e. "blue" suggests diseases in the liver; "red" corresponds to the heart; "yellow", the spleen; "white", the lung; and "black", the kidney.

These colours are also indicators of the nature of diseases:

The blue colour suggests diseases of wind, cold, pain, convulsion or blood stasis;

The red colour, caused by excessive filling of skin capillaries, suggests diseases of heat;

The yellow colour reveals dampness or blood deficiency;

The white colour indicates debility and the symptom-complex of cold;

The black colour suggests cold, pain, exhaustion or blood stasis.

Dark and gloomy complexion, hard to dispel, indicates disorder of internal organs, prolonged illness, or serious cases; while surficial lustre, clear and easy to dispel (vanish), indicates superficial illness (illness that has not attacked the vital organs), new diseases or minor cases.

3.1.2 Inspection of the tongue

In the clinical practice of Chinese medicine, the tongue is inspected as one of the indicators for diagnosis. The size, form, colour and moisture of the tongue proper and coating are the things to the examined.

3.1.2.1 The colour of the tongue

The normal tongue is pale red with a thin coating.

A whitish tongue (paler than normal) indicates deficiency of vital energy and blood.

A reddened tongue (redder than normal) indicates presence of heat. Deep redness of the tongue proper indicates presence of intense heat. A blue and purple tongue indicates blood stasis.

3.1.2.2 The coating of the tongue

White, thin and slippery coating of the tongue shows cold in the exterior.

White, slimy and greasy coating of the tongue, which is hard to wipe off, indicates presence of excessive phlegm and dampness or stagnancy of food.

Yellow, thick and slimy, dry coating of the tongue shows intense heat in the stomach.

Yellow but thin, slimy coating with white base shows that exterior pathogenic factors have penetrated into the interior.

Black and dry coating shows intense heat.

Black and moist coating shows intense cold.

Sometimes, the tongue is stained black by food or medicine, and this should be distinguished from its natural colour. Diagnosis cannot be based on such stained coating of the tongue.

3.1.2.3 The form of the tongue

Plum tongue indicates deficiency of vital function of the spleen and kidney.

Thin and shrunken tongue usually suggests deficiency of vital energy and blood, or interior heat.

Stiffness of the tongue shows block in the channels and collaterals, and is usually seen in cases of applexy or acute febrile disease.

Wry tongue, i.e. turning to one side while protruding, is seen in apoplexy.

Curled tongue shows exhaustion of the body fluid.

Tremor of the tongue shows heat in the interior and deficiency of the *Yin* (vital essence of the kidney).

3.1.2.4 The moisture of the tongue

A furless, smooth, mirror like tongue is usually seen in patients with deficiency of vital essence of the liver and kidney.

Prickly and dry tongue results from proliferation and

hypertrophy of taste buds, and it indicates intense heat in the viscera.

Blackish and moist tongue proper shows cold and pathogenic factors have reached the three *Yin* channels of both the hand and foot.

Black and dry coating shows interior heat and blood stasis.

When the colour of the tongue turns from grey to ashy black, or from pale purple to dark blue; or when a white, mildew-like coating appears, with rotten spots or looks like snow flakes; it means that the patient is dangerously ill, and death is impending.

3.2 Auscultation

Auscultation means audio-olfactive investigation. The physician listens to the patients' voice sounds of breath, cough, etc., which may serve to help differentiate the patients' symptom-complexes, and serve as a basis for the analysis and diagnosis of the cause, nature and location of the illness.

3.2.1 Voice

A feeble voice usually indicates a debilitated patient.

A loud voice may indicate a case of excessiveness.

If a patient speaks incoherently, it is most likely that he has lost consciousness.

Delirious speech usually occurs when a patient has high fever, especially when his central nervous system is attacked by evil wind.

3.2.2 Breathing

Heavy breathing often occurs with evil heat.

Stuffed nose and a heavy nasal sound often show a cold.

Heavy breathing with wheezing (a hissing sound from the throat) often indicates asthma caused by excessive phlegm.

3.2.3 Coughing

If one coughs with difficulty, it shows that the functional activities, including the respiratory function of the lung are impeded.

Low coughing, and little volume of the voice show insufficiency of vital energy or function of the spleen and stomach.

Loud snoring indicates partial blockage of the lung by phlegm and dampness.

Sudden coughing and cracking of the voice show excessiveness in the lung.

Prolonged coughing and loss of voice show deficiency of essence in the lung.

3.2.4 Belching

Sudden attack of a serious illness and persistent belching indicate intense pathological heat in the lung and stomach.

Prolonged illness and intermittent belching show deficiency of vital energy of the stomach.

3.2.5 Groaning

Groaning is often seen in cases of pains such as headache, stomach ache, general pain, pain in the waist, etc.

3.3 INTERROGATION

Interrogation means asking the patient questions about his illness to help with the diagnosis.

Zhang Jiebin 張介賓 (1553 — 1640), a doctor of the Ming Dynasty recommended ten areas of inquiry when making diagnosis: (1) chills and fever; (2) perspiration; (3) headache and general pains; (4) micturition and defecation; (5) appetite; (6) feeling in the chest and abdomen; (7) hearing; (8) thirst; (9) pulse taking and observation; (10) auscultation and smelling. Later people changed the last two areas into asking the patient about his old illnesses and causes of the new disease. Of woman patients inquiries should be made about menstration and leucorrhoea, and of children, measles.

The following is a detailed explanation of those areas.

3.3.1 Chills and fever

Chills and fever show exterior symptom-complexes, i.e. the human body is attacked by exogenous pathogenic factors.

In interior symptom-complex, i.e. the internal organ or the interior of the body is affected, chills and fever are not seen.

Aversion to cold and wind need not be a cold symptom-complex.

Fever need not indicate a heat symptom-complex.

Fever with aversion to cold, and headache or general pains, stiff neck, floating pulse, etc. is usually seen in *taiyangbing* (太陽病) — syndrome of the *yang* major channel, which lies on the surface of the body, due to attack of wind and cold on the surface of the body.

Fever, thirst, but without aversion to cold, indicate *yangmingbing* (陽明病) — syndrome of the splendid *yang* channel running within the interior of the body, such as influenza with illness in the intestines and stomach.

Alternate spells of fever and chills, with bitterness in the mouth and dry throat, indicate *shaoyangbing* (少陽病) — syndrome of the *yang* minor channel which runs between the exterior and interior of the body.

Intolerance of cold, without fever, but with cold limbs shows *yin* symptom-complex and deficiency of vital energy.

Hectic fever or tidal fever often indicates insufficiency symptom-complex.

3.3.2 Perspiration

Fever with perspiration is a sign of ·diseases caused by attacks of evil cold.

Acute febrile diseases may have the following symptoms:

fever, then perspiration, then heat clearing up, then fever coming back again, ...

Interior symptom-complex may be divided into deficiency of the *yang*, which is often seen with perspiration when awakening after sleep; and deficiency of the *yin* which is often seen with perspiration during sleep.

Cold limbs, hidden pulse, pale face and sweating incessantly usually indicate exhaustion.

3.3.3 Headache and general pains

Interrogation should include asking the patient how he feels.

Incessant headaches with cold and fever show cold in the exterior.

Intermittent headaches with dizziness show insufficiency symptom-complex.

Headaches together with general pains are often seen in influenza.

Pains in the joints, or travelling all over the body and limbs but no headache, are often seen in rheumatic fever.

Numb limbs indicate deficiency of vital energy.

Numbness in the thumbs and forefingers, or forearms, may be indications of apoplexy.

Abdominal pain with tenderness (the pain is aggravated when the abdomen is pressed) shows excessiveness symptom-complexes.

Abdominal pain which may be alleviated when the abdomen is pressed shows insufficiency symptom-complexes.

3.3.4 Defecation

A patient who suffers from constipation but still has normal appetite is suffering from constipation in *yang* nature.

When a patient eats less and less because of constipation, he is most likely suffering from constipation in *yin* nature.

Abdominal fullness and pain usually indicate excessiveness symptom-complexes.

Constipation without fullness and pain in the abdomen usually indicate insufficiency symptom-complexes.

Chronic constipation or that of the aged often indicates heat and dryness in the blood.

Bowels turning from dry to loose shows deficiency of vital energy in the Middle Burner (the spleen and the stomach).

Diarrhea with abdominal pain, and offensive smell from the stools are symptoms of indigestion caused by improper diet or overeating.

Tenesmus (an urgent desire for defecation but often ineffectual) indicates dysentery.

Watery diarrhea is usually caused by affection of cold.

Persistent diarrhea with vomiting may be an indication of acute gastroenteritis or cholera.

3.3.5 Micturition

Reddish brown urine shows heat symptom-complexes, caused by pathogenic heat or excessive vital function.

Clear and copious urine shows cold symptom-complexes, caused by cold factors or diminished vital function.

Turbid urine indicates febrile diseases caused by dampness and heat.

Frequent micturition with thirst indicates diabetes.

Dark yellow urine, with hematuresis and pain during micturition, indicate serious urination disturbance.

Incontinence of urine in the aged, or enuresis of infants often shows deficiency of *yin* (vital essence), *yang* (vital function) or *qi* (vital energy).

3.3.6 Appetite

A patient who has an excessive appetite usually has heat in the stomach.

One who eats little and has difficulty in digestion often has cold in the stomach.

Heat in the stomach is usually due to affection by evil heat or overeating of pungent and hot food. Other main symptoms are thirst, foul breath, preference for cold drinks, vomiting immediately after eating, etc.

Cold in the stomach is usually due to its insufficiency of vital function or caused by over-eating of raw and cold food. This is manifested by stomach pain relieved by warmth, vomiting in the evening food eaten in the morning, preference for hot drinks and food, etc.

Nausea and vomiting during early pregnancy are symptoms of morning sickness.

3.3.7 Chest and abdomen

Fullness in the chest usually indicates excessiveness symptom-complexes.

A depressed feeling in the chest usually indicates insufficiency symptom-complexes.

Restlessness shows heat symptom-complexes.

Masses or lumps in the abdomen show cold symptom-complexes.

A depressed feeling in the chest, which may be relieved with deep exhalation, shows stagnation of vital energy.

A stuffed feeling with sharp pain shows stasis of blood.

Shortness of breath with difficulty in breathing indicates deficiency of vital energy.

Chest pain with stuffiness may be seen with asthma, dyspnea and pain in the chest, which may radiate to the back.

3.3.8 Hearing

Sudden loss of hearing often appears in excessiveness symptom-complexes.

Chronic deafness or hardness of hearing shows insufficiency symptom-complexes.

Tinnitus (as if hearing the sound of blowing wind) shows illness caused by attack of wind and heat.

Tinnitus which is like the humming sound of a cicada usually shows illness of the liver or kidney.

A distended and painful feeling in the ear, with pus running out from the ear and difficulty in hearing, indicates attack of dampness and heat in the liver.

3.3.9 Thirst

Real thirst means that the patient feels thirsty and can drink. Pseudo-thirst means that he only feels thirsty but cannot drink or drinks very little.

Thirst with preference for cold drinks shows heat in the interior.

Thirst with preference for hot drinks shows cold in the interior.

Excessive thirst with normal micturition; a person who urinates twice as much as he drinks; or a person who urinates as much as he drinks show respectively three types of diabetes.

3.4 PALPATION

Palpation refers to pulse-taking. This was first recorded as a method for diagnosis in *Huangdi's Internal Classic* and *The Pulse Classic* (see Chapter 1).

When taking the pulse, the physician should be fully concentrated and very careful. He uses his index, middle and ring fingers to feel the patient's pulse by placing his fingers over the radial artery on the patient's wrist.

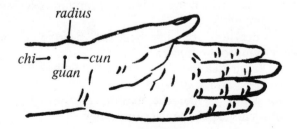

The three places for the three fingers are called *cun* (寸) (inch), *guan* (關) (bar), and *chi* (切) (cubit). The bar is just over the eminent head of the radius at the wrist, where the tip of the physician's middle finger should be placed. The inch is next to it on the distal side, where the tip of the index finger should rest. The cubit is on the proximal side of the bar, and it is where the ring finger is placed. (The physician should use his right hand to feel the pulse on the patient's right wrist, and vice versa. − Tr.)

The inch, bar and cubit on the left represent the pulse of the heart, the liver, and the kidney & small intestines respectively while those on the right represent the pulse of the lung, the spleen & stomach, and the bladder & large intestines.

When taking the pulse, the physician may have to use different manipulations such as lifting (resting the fingers on the wrist very lightly), pressing (feeling the pulse with proper force) and searching (varying the force or moving the fingers to get a more distinct pulse-reading).

3.4.1 Different kinds of pulses

There are all together twenty-eight kinds of pulses, which can be further divided into six categories in three pairs:

floating pulse and deep pulse, which respectively indicate the exterior symptom-complexes and interior symptom-complexes;

slow pulse and rapid pulse, which indicate the cold symptom-complexes and heat symptom-complexes;

smooth pulse and hesitant pulse, which indicate the insufficiency symptom-complexes and excessiveness symptom-complexes.

3.4.1.1 Floating pulse (*fumai*) (浮脈)

Floating pulse can be felt by light touch and grows faint on hard pressure, seen usually in the initial stage of diseases, indicating the exterior of the body is affected.

Floating but hard and hollow pulse *(gemai)* (革脈), which is like the feeling of the surface of a drum, indicates loss of blood.

Floating and soft (superficial and fine) which can be felt on light pressure but grows faint on hard pressure (called *rumai* (濡脈) in Chinese) is seen in cases with deficiency of blood and vital essence.

3.4.1.2 Deep pulse *(chenmai)* (沉脈)

Deep pulse can only be felt while pressing hard. It shows that disease is located in the interior of the body.

Deep pulse also includes hidden pulse *(fumai* (伏脈); a different word in Chinese — Tr.), which can only be felt on strong pressure and seen in cases of syncope, shock, severe pain, etc.

Firm pulse (*laomai* (牢脈)), a forceful and taut pulse, felt only by hard pressure, can usually be seen in cases with accumulation of cold factor such as formation of firm masses.

Weak pulse (*ruomai* (弱脈)) means soft, weak pulse which can only be felt by hard pressure, and seen in cases of general debility.

A pulse felt forceful on both light and heavy pressure is called *shimai* (實脈) — replete or forceful pulse, which is seen in excessiveness symptom-complexes with undamaged body resistance.

A pulse, felt feeble and as though avoiding the physician's finger, is called *xumai* (虛脈) — feeble pulse, seen in cases of debility.

Hollow pulse (*konmai* (孔脈), floating, large and empty inside, felt like a scallion stalk, is seen in cases with massive loss of blood.

To sum up, deep or floating pulses are differentiated from the force of the pulse, which is felt by the physician.

3.4.1.3 Slow pulse *(chimai)* (遲脈)

Slow or retarded pulse, with less than four beats to one cycle of respiration (or less than 60 beats per minute), usually indicates cold symptom-complexes.

The Chinese term *huanmai* (緩脈) refers to "moderate pulse", which has usually four beats to one cycle of respiration with even rhythm and moderate tension. It usually indicates recovery of a patient, such as when the fever is removed after perspiration and the patient has returned to normal condition.

Slow and uneven pulse (*jiemai*) (結脈), which pauses at irregular intervals, is often seen in cases caused by attacks of dampness and cold.

3.4.1.4 Rapid or frequent pulse *(shumai)* (數脈)

Rapid or frequent pulse has more than five beats to one cycle of respiration (or more than 90 beats per minute). It indicates presence of heat.

Tremulous pulse (*dongmai*) (動脈) refers to quick and jerking pulse, which can be felt at the bar only (it can not be felt at the inch or cubit). It is seen in cases with pain or being frightened, or in pregnant women.

Swift pulse (*jimai*) (疾脈), over seven to eight beats to one cycle of respiration or 120 – 140 beats per minute, is seen in febrile diseases with high fever or advanced cases of consumption.

Running pulse (*cumai*) (促脈), rapid with irregular intermittence, is usually seen in cases with excessive heat and stagnation of vital energy, blood and phlegm.

Intermittent pulse (*daimai*) (代脈) pausing at regular intervals, indicates the feeble condition of the viscera.

Scattered pulse (*sanmai*) (散脈), a pulse diffusing on light touch and faint on hard pressure, is seen in critical cases and shows insufficiency of original vital energy.

The slow pulses and the rapid pulses are distinguished mainly according to the frequency of the pulse — the times of beating in one cycle of respiration. It is obvious to see the differences.

3.4.1.5 Smooth or slippery pulse *(huamai)* (滑脈)

Smooth or slippery pulse means a pulse beating like beads rolling on a plate, seen in patients with dampness or stagnation of food, and also in pregnant women. This kind of pulse may be seen in some normal persons.

Taut pulse (*xianmai*) (弦脈), a pulse beating like a tremulous music string, is seen usually in malaria or cases with liver trouble or severe pains.

Tense pulse (*jinmai*) (緊脈), felt like a tightly stretched cord, is often seen in cases with exterior or interior cold.

Long pulse (*changmai*) (長脈) refers to a pulse with large extent and prolonged strokes. This kind of pulse is observed in cases where confrontation between the body resistance and invading factors is going on hard.

Full pulse (*hongmai*) (洪脈), a pulse beating like dashing waves forceful rising and gradual declining, is seen usually in cases with excessive evil heat.

3.4.1.6 Hesitant pulse *(semai)* (澀脈)

Hesitant pulse is a pulse with small, fine, slow joggling tempo like scraping bamboo with knife. It indicates sluggishness of blood circulation caused by deficiency of blood and essence or stagnancy of vital energy and blood.

Short pulse (*duanmai*) (短脈), a pulse with short extent, easily to be felt at the cubit, yet not obvious while felt at the inch and bar, strikes the middle finger sharply and leaves it quickly. Such pulse shows stagnancy or deficiency of vital energy.

Faint pulse (*weimai*) (微脈), a thready and soft pulse which is scarcely perceptible, shows exhaustion of vital energy to the extreme.

Fine or thready pulse (*ximai*) (細脈), a pulse as thin as a silk thread, feeble yet always perceptible on hard pressure, indicates exhaustion of blood.

The physician can tell the difference between smooth and hesitant pulses by the smooth or puckery feel.

Pulse-reading is a very complicated matter and depends largely on the physician's skill and experience. In making a diagnosis, the physician should take into account both the pulse condition and the symptoms and signs observed with other methods, so as to penetrate phenomena and grasp the reality.

3.4.2 Multi-feature pulses

Abnormal pulse can indicate very complicated cases when it shows two or more distinct features. This kind of pulse is called multi-feature pulse.

The following are a few examples of different multi-feature pulses:

3.4.2.1 Different kinds of multi-featured floating pulses

Floating pulse mainly indicates exterior symptom-complexes.

Floating and loose pulse shows a cold.

Floating and tense pulse shows febrile diseases.

Floating and slippery pulse shows stagnation of phlegm and food.

Floating and feeble pulse shows affection due to seasonal pathogenic factors in the summer.

Floating and hollow pulse shows hemorrhage.

Floating and rapid pulse shows illness caused by attack of wind and heat.

Floating and full pulse shows mania.

3.4.2.2 Multi-features with deep-pulse

Deep pulse mainly indicates interior symptom-complexes. Deep and fine pulse shows deficiency of vital energy in liver and kidney.

Deep and slow pulse shows chronic cold, and cold in the kidney.

Deep and slippery pulse shows stagnation of food, or retention of phlegm and fluid.

Deep and hidden pulse shows acute gastroenteritis.

Deep and rapid pulse shows heat in the interior.

Deep and tense pulse shows cold in the interior.

Deep and taut pulse shows disturbance due to perverted function of the liver.

3.4.2.3 Multi-features with slow pulse

Slow pulse mainly indicates cold symptom-complex.

Slow and floating pulse shows deficiency of vital energy.

Slow and deep pulse shows cold in the interior.

Slow and hesitant pulse shows deficiency of blood.

Slow and loose pulse shows affection of cold and dampness.

Slow and slippery pulse shows arthralgia due to wind and phlegm.

Slow and fine pulse shows contraction.

3.4.2.4 Rapid pulse with other features

Rapid pulse mainly indicates heat symptom-complex.

Rapid and slippery pulse shows heat symptoms caused by excessive pathogenic factors while the body resistance is still sufficient.

Rapid and fine pulse shows interior heat with deficiency of vital essence, chiefly referred to that of the kidney.

Rapid and floating pulse shows fever caused by exogenous pathogenic factors.

Rapid and deep pulse shows interior heat.

3.4.2.5 Multi-feature with slippery pulse

Slippery pulse mainly indicates excessive symptom-complexes.

Slippery, floating pulse shows that the patient has phlegm caused by the attack of wind.

Slippery, deep pulse shows stagnation of phlegm and food.

Slippery, gigantic pulse is seen in cases with excessive heat in the stomach.

3.4.2.6 Hesitant pulse showing other features

Hesitant pulse indicates deficiency symptom-complex.

Hesitant and floating pulse shows insufficiency in the exterior.

Hesitant and deep pulse shows insufficiency in the interior.

Hesitant and weak pulse shows impairment of body fluid, especially of the lung and stomach.

Besides the above-mentioned 28 kinds of pulses, there are seven others indicating inpending death, such as "shrimp-darting pulse", a nearly imperceptible pulse with occasional darting beats; "dripping pulse", an extremely retarded pulse resembling water dripping from a roof crack; "boiling pulse", an extremely floating and rapid pulse like bubbles rising to the surface in boiling water; etc. They are all death indicators. Therefore, there is no need for detailed discussion.

Chapter 4

Causes of Diseases

According to an ancient classification of aetiology, there are three categories of pathogeny: Exogenous, endogenous and non-exo-endogenous.

Exogenous causes of disease refer chiefly to the excessive and sudden changes of weather. Endogenous causes refer to excessive emotional changes. The third category, non-exo-endogenous causes, means causes related neither to external nor to internal influences, such as intemperance in eating, drinking and sexual life, overwork, etc.

The ancient people summed up the weather changes as six atmospheric influences to the human body: wind, cold, summer heat, dampness, dryness and fire. Under normal circumstances, man can cope with these influences and will not fall ill. The sudden and abnormal weather changes give rise to various diseases.

4.1 WIND AND COLD

Wind and cold are causes of disease. Medical classics described wind as the first and foremost factor to cause various diseases. Here, wind does not exclusively refer to the air in motion as the result of natural forces. There are external wind (natural wind) which causes frostbite and flu, and internal wind, a pathological change due to excessive heat or deficiency of blood or vital essence marked by dizziness, fainting, tremor, facial paralysis, etc.

4.2 SUMMER HEAT AND DAMPNESS

Summer heat brings on symptoms such as fever, headache, thirst, restlessness, sweating, rapid gigantic pulse.

Dampness, also related to summer, causes many diseases such as rheumatism. It can also give rise to stomach trouble, dropsy, athlete's foot, whites, eczema, etc.

There is endogenous dampness and exogenous dampness, the former referring to stagnancy of water within the body caused by deficient function of the stomach and intestines, manifested by loss of appetite, diarrhea, scanty urine, sallow face, etc., and the latter means a pathogenic factor attacking a victim living and working in damp places, bringing on symptoms such as headache, lassitude, heaviness in the limbs, fullness in the chest, joint pains, etc.

4.3 DRYNESS AND FIRE

Both dryness and fire are pathogenic factors. Dryness impairs body fluid and sometimes is caused by the seven emotional factors: joy, anger, melancholy, anxiety, sorrow, fear and fright. These are reactions of the human body to the outside world and do not usually lead to disease. But if in excess, they may lead to abnormal function of the internal organs and derangement of vital energy and blood, hence disease.

There is internal and external dryness: the former is caused by the lack of body fluid and manifested by restlessness and thirst; the latter is caused by undernourishment and manifested by dry skin.

4.4 INTERNAL INJURY

Internal injury refers to diseases caused by emotional strains, improper diet, overwork, sexual intemperance, etc.

Intemperance in sexual life as well as marrying too early and bearing too many children will lead to lumbago, seminal emission, dizziness and impairment of the reproductive essence stored in the kidney. It is also believed that over fatigue and over strain may impair the spleen and the original vital energy.

The understanding of the causes of diseases can not only help us cure diseases but also prevent them. Chinese traditional medicine attaches importance to the "struggle between the patients' resistance and the invading pathogenic factors." If the former can overcome the latter, diseases can be cured. On the contrary, if the latter defeats the former, the patient will go from bad to worse and even die. The theory also holds that physical training, proper diet and balance between work and rest can build up one's resistance and a balance inside his body and helps him achieve health.

Chapter 5

Principles of Treatment and Differentiation of Symptom-Complexes

The medical classic "Plain Questions" argues that the principles of treatment should be based on the conception of the organism as a whole, and an overall analysis of symptoms and signs. According to this theory, stress should be put in treating the fundamental cause, importance attached to the internal causes of the human body and the relations between the patient's resistance and the invading pathogenic factors and what is primary differentiated from what is secondary.

5.1 INCIDENTAL AND FUNDAMENTAL, GREATER AND LESSER URGENCY

"To treat a disease one should find out its root or cause" is the principle put forward by the "Plain Questions", meaning the proper measure should be taken according to the actual conditions of the genuine energy (body resistance) of the human body.

According to the basic theories of traditional Chinese medicine, "the fundamental" refers to the root or cause of a disease, primary onset of a disease and disease in the interior while "the incidental" refers to manifestation of a disease in the exterior. Either the fundamental or the incidental aspect of the disease can be treated first. Generally speaking, in emergency cases treat the acute symptoms first, when these have been relieved, treat their fundamental cause.

Usually, the genuine energy of the human body is the fundamental and one should pay attention to the patient's resistance to disease. However, if the patient's genuine energy is not yet impaired, but the invading pathogenic factors are acute, the latter should be treated first. Again, in cases of haemorrhage, treatment should be given after finding out the cause. But if massive haemorrhage endangers the patient's life, measures to stop bleeding should be regarded as most urgent.

The relations of the fundamental and incidental are by no means immutable. A patient may first have a headache and then a fever. Both are symptoms and it is hard to say which is fundamental or incidental. Judgement should be made according to the actual conditions.

5.2 ADJUSTING *YIN* AND *YANG*

According to the theories of traditional Chinese medicine, imbalance of *Yin* and *Yang* is the root of disease. Hence adjusting *Yin* and *Yang* is the starting point of treating the fundamental aspect of the disease.

Yin and *Yang* are a philosophical concept used in ancient times to interpret everything in the universe. It began to be applied to medicine in the Spring and Autumn Period (770-476 B.C.).

In medicine, *Yin* and *Yang* mean different things. While referring to various antitheses in anatomy, Bowels are *Yang* while Viscera are *Yin*; vital energy is *Yang* while blood is *Yin*; and the back is *Yang* while abdomen is *Yin*. In physiology and pathology, the concept of *Yin* (blood) and *Yang* (vital energy) are also used. Both exogenous pathogenic factors of *Yin* nature or the weakening of the *yang* vital energy can present themselves as cold symptom-complex. Again, pathogenic factors of *yang* nature or the impairment of the *yin* body fluid may be manifested as heat symptom-complex. An illness of heat nature in the extreme may show symptoms and signs of cold nature. This is called the transformation of *yin* and *yang* into each other under certain conditions.

The theory of *yin* and *yang* can be applied to diagnosis and treatment. Heat of the *yang* nature can be checked by reinforcing the *yin* (vital essence), and cold of the *yin* nature can be checked by replenishing the *yang* (vital function). This method is called "the interaction of *yin* and *yang*." The theory is also used to differentiate the function of different medicines. Drugs for clearing up internal cold or sudorifics are called *yang* while those for dispelling internal heat called *yin*. Treating the fundamental aspect of a disease means adjustment of *yin* and *yang*. Exuberance of *yang* or *yin* or deficiency of both *yin* and *yang*, according to the theory, should be adjusted by reinforcing *yang, yin* or both, respectively.

5.3 DIFFERENCE OF SYMPTOMS AND THEIR TRANSFORMATION

Symptoms of a disease are changeable under different conditions. Therefore one should analyse the particularity and universality of the causes and mechanisms of diseases, in connection with different season, location and environment, seeking differences from similarities and similarities from differences. The same disease may have different symptoms and different diseases may have the same symptoms. Therefore, different methods of treatment can be applied to the same kind of disease in the light of different physical reactions and clinical manifestations. Likewise, one can treat different diseases by the same method if they are alike in clinical manifestations and pathogeny.

Bronchial asthma, for instance, can be analysed from different syndromes: exterior and interior, heat and cold, insufficiency (or deficiency) and excessiveness. The methods of treatment include dispelling pathogenic factors from the exterior of the body by diaphoresis, ventilating and smoothing the troubled lung, or resolving phlegm with warm properties, etc.

Chronic enteritis, prolapse of the anus and uterus are different diseases, but they are caused by the sinking of vital energy of the Middle Burner (the spleen), so the same method — reinforcing the Middle Burner and replenishing the vital energy — can be used.

Symptoms constantly change. Exterior symptom-complex and interior symptom-complex are interchangeable, so are excessiveness symptom-complex and insufficiency symptom-complex, and heat symptom-complex and cold symptom-complex. A patient may feel cold and have a fever — symptom of cold in the exterior. The next day, he no longer feels cold, but fever remains, indicating he is suffering from heat in the interior. In cases of infectious febrile diseases due to exogenous pathogenic factors, some patients may have a fever first accompanied with coughing and pain in the chest — exterior heat symptoms. But he may then sweat too much, have cold limbs and deep and fine pulse, which indicates a deficiency in the interior. So the doctors must pay keen attention to the changing symptoms in order to choose the right medicine.

5.4 CONSIDERATION OF MEDICAL TREATMENT BASED ON VARIOUS CONDITIONS

There is a variety of methods of treatment. But in applying

these methods, one has to consider climatic and seasonal conditions, geographical localities and the patient's constitution. There is no same pattern to follow.

The doctors may treat a disease in a routine and regular way, or by reverse process. They may also combine external treatment with tonifying drugs in favor of discharging pus. Treating the disease in a routine and regular way means to use therapy and drugs opposite in nature to the disease — treating cold symptom-complex with drugs warm or hot in proper, and vice versa; treating deficiency symptom-complex with reinforcing or replenishing method while treating excessiveness with method of purgation and reduction.

Treating full conditions with filling method and "open" conditions with "opening" methods are methods by reverse process. Here are two cases to show these methods:

— Diarrhea accompanied by stomach pain, slimy and greasy coating of the tongue and slippery pulse, is caused by food stagnancy in the stomach and intestine. In this case, the purgation method — to clear stagnation — can be used. This is also called treating "open" conditions with "opening" methods.

— Distension of abdomen, accompanied by loss of appetite, pale tongue and feeble pulse, is caused by deficiency in the spleen which leads to syndrome of the Middle Burner. In this case, medicine should be taken to reinforce the vital energy and the function of the spleen. This is called treating full conditions with filling method.

As for affection of both the exterior and interior of the body, medicines should dispel pathogenic factors from both.

As for a patient whose resistance is declining and illness is developing, medicines should drive out invading pathogenic agents and reinforce the body resistance at the same time.

In using medicines, different conditions of the patients should be taken into consideration. For old and weak patients, doctors must be very careful in using purgatives to clear stagnation of food and relieve water retention. In the

North, and for patients with good physical conditions, *Mahuang* (Herba Ephedrae) and *Guizhi* (Ramulus Cinnamomi) can be used to promote eruption in measles. But in the South, and for weak patients, *Jingjie* (Herba Schizonepetae), *Bohe* (Herba Menthae) and similar herbs should be used instead for the same purpose.

Chapter 6

Eight Methods of Treatment

Diaphoresis, emesis, purgation, mediation, febrifugal, warming, elimination and tonification are the eight therapeutic methods used by the Chinese traditional medicine.

The methods were first summed up in *Medicine Comprehended (Yixue Xinwu),* a concise and practical work written by Chang Guopeng, a celebrated physician of the Qing Dynasty. Apart from listing different methods of treatment, the book explains the dialectical relations between heat and cold, insufficiency and excessiveness, exterior and interior, and *yin* and *yang*, of the disease. Included in the book are febrile diseases, miscellaneous diseases, gynecological diseases, surgical lesions, as well as diseases of eye, ear, nose, mouth and throat. Essentials of the eight methods follow:

6.1 DIAPHORETIC METHOD

All means that induce perspiration by drugs fall into this category, which was first recorded in the *Huangdi's Internal Classic.* Diaphoretics are used in treating exterior symptom-complex such as chills, headache, common cold, etc.

There are two ways to induce perspiration by drugs. The

first way is to combine diaphoretics with an excitant, such as the Decoction of Ephedra and Decoction of Cinnamon Twigs.

The Decoction of Ephedra consists of *Mahuang* (Herba Ephedrae), *Guizhi* (Ramulus Cinnamomi), *Xingren* (Semen Armeniacae Amarum) and *Gancao* (Radix Glycyrrhizae). This decoction can dispel pathogenic factors from the exterior of the body, promote the function of a troubled lung and relieve cough and therefore is used for treating cold, fever, asthmatic symptoms, headache, blockage of sweat glands, and pain in the arms and legs.

The Decoction of Cinnamon Twigs consists of *Guizhi, Baishao* (Radix Paeoniae Alba), *Shengjiang* (Rhizoma Zingiberis), *Gancao* and *Dazao* (Fructus Ziziphi Jujubae). It can dispel pathogenic factors from the superficial muscles and rectify derangement of defensive and constructive energy and therefore is effective in treating cold, fever, headache, aversion to wind, stuffed and running nose, and floating and loose pulse. The decoction can also be applied to some miscellaneous internal diseases caused by derangement of defensive and constructive energy marked by alternate spells of fever and chills, spontaneous sweating and aversion to wind.

The second way to induce perspiration is combined with bringing down a fever — diaphoretics with antipyretics. The powder of Lonicera and Forsythia, as a diaphoretic with drugs pungent in flavour and cooling in property, belongs to this category. The powder consists of *Jinyinhua* (Flos Lonicerae), *Lianqiao* (Fructus Forsythiae), *Niubangzi* (Fructus Arctii), *Bohe* (Herba Menthae), *Jingjie* (Herba Schizonepetae), *Douzhi* (Semen Sajae Praeparatum), *Danzhuye* (Herba Lophatheri), *Lugen* (Rhizoma Phragmitis), *Gancao,* and *Jiegeng* (Radix Platycodi).

The powder is used for the early stage of influenza marked by fever without aversion to cold, marked also by no sweating or difficult sweating, headache, thirst, sore throat, cough, etc. Pills made of the same recipe are available.

In using diaphoretics, attention must be paid to the following:

(1) In dispelling pathogenic heat, too much perspiration must be prevented because too much perspiration is apt to affect the heart and lead to thirst and restlessness.

(2) It is not appropriate to use this method for those who suffer from anaemia, ulcer or a feeble heart. If they have to take diaphoretics, they must at the same time take tonics or refrigerants.

(3) After taking diaphoretics, one must keep himself warm and drink plenty of hot water.

6.2 EMETIC METHOD

Emetic method means to expel noxious substances with emetics or mechanical stimulation to induce vomiting. The method is used when phlegm blocks the throat and interrupts breathing or when stagnant food causes abdominal distension and pain or when poisonous substance accidently eaten is still in the stomach.

Emetics include *Erchen Decoction,* which has the following ingredients: *Chenpi* (Pericarpium Titri Reticulatae), *Banxia* (Rhizoma Pinelliae Praeparata), *Fuling* (Poria) and *Gancao* (Radix Glyeyrrhizae Praparata).

Emetics also include the stem of melons, gourd, black false hellebore and Chalcanthile, etc. Goose or duck feathers can be used to stimulate the throat.

Fragile people and pregnant women are not advised to use this method.

6.3 PURGATION METHOD

An old saying goes like this: "Diaphoresis is used to treat

external diseases and purgation is used for internal ones." Purgation is to relieve constipation in order to preserve *yin* fluid, which refers to all kinds of nutrient fluid in the body especially that of the viscera. The Drastic Purgative Decoction (see Chapter 8, 8.1) is effective in treating syndrome with the bowels involved, marked by fever, constipation, abdominal pain with tenderness, yellow and thick fur of the tongue, slippery and full pulse.

Generally speaking, purgation is used to relieve stagnant matter in the intestines. The method is not appropriate for insufficiency and cold. It is only for those who are strong enough to stand it and for excessive symptom-complex.

There are two kinds of purgatives: drugs of cold nature such as *Dahuang* (Rhubarb), and those with warm nature like *Badou* (Croton seed).

Purgation should not be applied to weak people and pregnant women because it might cause exhaustion or hiccup.

6.4 MEDIATION METHOD

First mentioned in the classic *Treatise on Febrile Diseases* more than 2,000 years ago, Mediation is used to treat affection located between the exterior and interior with symptom-complex marked by alternate fever and chills, fullness and choking feeling in the chest and costal regions, bitter taste in the mouth, dry throat, nausea and loss of appetite.

The Mild Decoction of Bupleurum (consisting of *Chaihu* (Radix Bupleuri), *Huang qin* (Radix Scutellariae), *Dazao* (Fructus Ziziphi Jujubae), *Shengjiang* (Rhizoma Zingiberis Recens), *Banxia* (Rhizoma Pinelliae Praeparata), *Gancao* (Radix Glycyrrhizae), *Dangshen* (Radix Codonopsis Pilosulae), an outstanding recipe in this category, is effective in treating fullness and tightness in the chest and costal regions, fidget and nausea, by regulating the correlations of viscera, channels, vital energy and blood, removing pathogenic factors and restoring normal functions.

There are various ways of mediation, with emphasis on clearing up heat, removing stagnation of food and other matters, dispelling internal cold, reinforcing vital energy, etc.

The method should not be understood as mediation at will. To use the method at random may have bad consequences.

6.5 FEBRIFUGAL METHOD

The method is used to treat acute febrile diseases and other diseases with internal heat. Heat symptom-complex is extremely complicated and there are great differences between heat in the exterior and in the interior. For the heat in the interior, there are syndrome of the secondary defensive system and syndrome of the blood system. Therefore, one must be very careful in differentiating various symptoms before using the drugs. The method can only be applied to those febrile diseases marked by thirst without aversion to cold.

Another thing to remember is that one should not take febrifuges for long. Otherwise they will injure the spleen and stomach and feeble people and pregnant women should not take febrifuges even if they suffer from febrile diseases.

Some heat syndromes which are not caused by pathogenic heat can be treated by drugs hot in property. This method is called "leading heat to its root."

6.6 WARMING METHOD

Just opposite to the febrifugal method, warming method is used to treat cold symptom-complex marked by intolerance of cold and wind, cold limbs, spontaneous sweating, sudden pain in the abdomen, breathlessness and frequent micturition, etc.

Employed for excitation and in the treatment of emergency and in restoration of vital function from collapse, the method is designed usually for fragile people.

It is not applicable to heat symptom-complex because it may cause haematemesis.

Both febrifugal and warming methods can be effective only when they are co-ordinated with the principles of treatment and in keeping with the actual conditions of the patient.

6.7 ELIMINATION METHOD

The method is used for treating goiter, dyspepsia, gathering and brewing of dampness and heat in the body, and similar diseases. The drugs used can remove stagnancy of food, disintegrate masses formed by stagnated vital energy and blood, etc. *Cigu* (arrowhead), *kunbu* (Laminaria) and *ezhu* (Rhizoma Zedoariae), for instance, can soften and remove stagnated food and blood stasis.

The method is not good for emergency cases, nor for very weak people.

The use of drugs to drive out invading pathogenic agents cost blood and vital energy and therefore they must not be over-used. The same is true with elimination method. Usually, patients should first take laxatives and after some time use tonics.

6.8 TONIFYING METHOD

As the *Internal Classic* put it, "Deficiency symptom-complex should be treated with reinforcing or replenishing method." By using tonics, the method is designed to treat the deficiency of vital energy, blood, vital function and essence of the body.

There are three kinds of reinforcement: warm reinforcement for deficiency of *yang* (vital function) usually accompanied with cold symptoms; febrifugal reinforcement for deficiency of *yin* (vital essence) associated with production of internal heat; and normal reinforcement for general deficiency symptom-complex.

While using tonifying method, one must take care of the spleen and the stomach which "provide the material basis of the acquired constitution," as one ancient classic put it. No tonic is useful to the body if spleen and stomach go wrong.

The method is not applicable to affection due to exogenous pathogenic factor because, using the method in that case is just like "keeping a thief inside by closing the door."

So much for the essentials of the eight methods. It must be pointed out that none of these should be isolated out. They are effective only when they are used in a comprehensive way on the basis of an overall analysis of symptoms and signs.

Chapter 7
Eight Principal Syndromes

The traditional Chinese medicine analyses and differentiates pathological conditions in accordance with the eight principal syndromes, i.e., *yin* and *yang,* exterior and interior, heat and cold, insufficiency (or deficiency) and excessiveness.

In his complete works appearing in 1624 A.D., the medical man Zhang Jiebin (about 1563 — 1640) explained that to examine *yin* and *yang* first is the guiding principle of the healing art; and relations between exterior and interior, heat and cold, insufficiency and excessiveness are the key of medical knowledge.

The clinical practice of the traditional Chinese medicine stresses the differentiation of symptom-complexes. The method of treatment and using of drugs are decided on the basis of an analysis of the syndromes.

According to the theory, exterior and interior, heat and cold, insufficiency and excessiveness are both opposite and complementary to each other. Their relationship can be described by the concept of *yin* and *yang.*

The breakdown of balanced equilibrium of *yin* and *yang* and the confrontation between the body resistance and pathogenic factors are two main elements in deciding the nature of a disease.

The human body is an organic whole and is at the same

time divided into two opposites — *yin* and *yang,* the imbalance of which is the root cause of disease.

For instance, in the process of breathing, the lung on the one hand keeps the pathway of air unobstructed and disseminates vital energy throughout and on the other hand, it cleans the inspired air and keeps it and the vital energy flowing downward. The two functions are a pair of contradictions. If either function is impeded, diseases may occur.

The lung and kidney are also opposite to each other in breathing. The lung performs the function of respiration and the kidney has the function of controlling and promoting inspiration. If they fail to do so, disease occurs.

Traditional Chinese medicine attaches great importance to observing the patient's complexion which is an outward manifestation of vital energy. White colour of the complexion usually indicates presence of deficiency of blood and vital energy and redness suggests deficiency of vital essence and heat in the interior.

7.1 EXTERIOR AND INTERIOR

The human body is composed of Exterior and Interior. The former consists of skin, sweat glands of the surface layer and muscle, etc. The latter includes heart, brains, lung, kidney, stomach, intestines.

These are also exterior and interior symptom-complexes. The former refers to the symptoms caused by the attack of exogenous pathogenic factors on the external part of the human body and respiratory tract. Although the cause is the same, exterior symptom-complex includes cold and heat syndromes. Cold in the exterior is marked by chilliness, fever, headache, general aching, stuffy nose and cough, as well as a floating and tense pulse. Heat in the exterior is marked by fever (but no chills), sore throat, thirst, yellow phlegm, and floating and rapid pulse, etc.

Interior symptom-complex indicates the development or transmission of a disease from the exterior to the interior of the body, or derangement of functions of the internal organs because of over eating, over fatigue or excessive emotional changes. There are many kinds of interior symptom-complexes. Deficiency in the interior is marked by pale look, vomiting, brown urine, palpitation and insomnia. Excessiveness in the interior is marked by abdominal distension and pain, constipation, hectic fever and delirium.

The concept of interior and exterior tells a doctor where the disease comes from and how it may develop. If a patient has headache, general pain and fear of cold first and then has a fever and feels restless, his disease has been transmitted from the exterior to the interior of the body. That is why the observation of interior and exterior plays an important role in diagnosis.

7.2 COLD AND HEAT

The doctor of Chinese medicine first differentiates cold and heat, the two main features of an illness, in diagnosis.

The cold symptom-complex is caused by cold factor or diminished vital function. Heat symptom-complex is caused by pathogenic heat or excessive vital function, or by heat transmitted from cold factor.

Cold symptom-complex is an expression of the drop of body temperature and the falling of organic functions caused by certain stimulation. Heat symptom-complex is an indication of the going up of temperature and hyperfunction of organism.

Generally speaking, both cold and heat symptom-complexes have different features. For instance, the patient of cold syndrome has a preference for hot drinks and food, and does not feel thirsty. He usually has a whitish and slippery coat on the tongue. On the contrary, a patient with heat syndrome is fond of cold drinks and food, and is marked by constipation, hectic fever and yellow and prickly coating of the tongue.

However, heat syndrome is sometimes marked by loose bowels and cold limbs and cold syndrome is marked by hectic fever and constipation. There are cases of cold showing pseudo-heat symptoms or heat showing pseudo-cold symptoms. So if one fails to analyse symptoms in a comprehensive way, he is apt to make mistakes in treatment.

7.3 DEFICIENCY AND EXCESSIVENESS

Deficiency symptom-complex refers to the weakening of body resistance caused by the lack of vital substance (chiefly from food essence).

Excessiveness symptom-complex is caused by exogenous pathogenic factors or by accumulation of pathologic products due to dysfunction of internal organs, such as phlegm, stagnant blood and food, etc. As the classic *Plain Questions* (see Chapter 1) put it, "symptom-complexes of excessiveness occur when pathogenic factors are in abundance; symptom-complexes of insufficiency occur when the patient's vital essence and energy are severely damaged."

Deficiency is marked by pallor, fatigue, palpitation, shortness of breath, spontaneous sweat, etc.

Excessiveness is marked by reddish face, heavy breathing, phlegm retention, dyspnea and abdominal pain, etc.

The doctor usually differentiates deficiency and excessiveness syndromes by deciding whether the patient sweats and has fullness sensation in the abdomen and whether his pulse is forceful or not.

In short, these two syndromes indicate the physical condition of a patient and the state of exogenous pathogenic factors. Generally speaking, deficiency is often connected with prolonged illness and old people while excessiveness usually has to do with new illness and people in their prime.

7.4 *YIN* AND *YANG*

The *yin* symptom-complex is often marked by cold limbs fondness of warmth, debility and depression. Syndromes of cold and deficiency generally belong to this category.

Manifested by hot body, fondness of cool, hyperactivity, excitability, heavy breathing and cracked lips, the *yang* symptom-complex usually refers to syndromes of heat and excessiveness.

Yin and *yang*, as this book has previously explained, are an ancient philosophical concept which refers to the attribute of things rather than to the things themselves. In *Huangdi's Internal Classic*, the concept, which describes two things as being both opposite and complementary to each other, was applied to explain contradictions in the medical field, forming the theoretical basis for the traditional Chinese medicine.

In the Han Dynasty, Zhang Zhongjing used the theory of *yin* and *yang* and developed therapeutic methods of diaphoresis, emesis, purgation, mediation, invigoration, heat reduction for treating febrile diseases in the influential *Treatise on Febrile Diseases*, initiating diagnosis and treatment based on an overall analysis of symptoms and signs.

The above four pairs of syndromes condition each other. Usually, diseases are caused by excess of either *yin* and *yang*, or by deficiency of either *yin* and *yang*. When a balance is achieved between excess and deficiency, illness disappears.

To restore the balanced equilibrium of *yin* and *yang* is the aim of medical treatment as well as that of physical training.

Chapter 8

Seven Prescriptions

Prescriptions or recipes, an important part of traditional Chinese medicine, have long been recorded by ancient medical classics. There are seven kinds of recipes in Chinese materia medica: major (heavy), minor (mild), slow-acting, quick-acting, recipes with one or more principal ingredients and compound recipes.

A recipe usually consists of many different medicinal substances. Compared with a single drug, recipes have at least three advantages:

1) A recipe can be used in comprehensive treatment while a single drug is usually effective only to one symptom;

2) Usually the more efficacious a drug is, the more side effects it produces. The combination of various ingredients in a recipe can produce desired therapeutic effect in unison and reduce toxic or side effects;

3) The number of the ingredients in a recipe can be increased or decreased according to symptoms while a single drug has little leeway.

A recipe usually contains the principal, adjuvant, auxiliary and conductant ingredients. According to the theory of Chinese medicine, the principal ingredient provides the principal curative action; the adjuvant helps strengthen the principal action; the auxiliary and correctant ingredient relieves secondary symptoms or tempers the action of the principal ingredient when the latter is too potent; and the conductant directs action to the affected channel or site.

The ingredients in a recipe are by no means immutable. The composition of ingredients in a prescription is decided by the complicated causes and symptoms of diseases.

8.1 HEAVY AND MILD RECIPES

A heavy recipe which consists of big dosage of ingredients is made for major diseases while mild recipe, with small dosage, is for minor illness.

A doctor should not hesitate to use a heavy recipe if that is the way to save a patient from crucial diseases. Hesitation can only worsen the disease and even leads to the death of the patient.

The Drastic Purgative Decoction (*Da Chengqi Tang*) is a heavy recipe. Consisting of *dahuang* (Radix et Rhisoma Rhei), *mangxiao* (Natril Suljas), *zhishi* (Fructus Aurantii Immaturus), and *houpo* (Cortex Magnoliae Officinalis), it is used to purge the bowels of accumulated waste matter and internal heat. Syndromes to which the recipe is effective include fever, dilirious speech, abdominal pain with tenderness, constipation, etc. It is also used for acute appendicitis.

Heavy recipes are not used for minor illness, nor when pathogenic factors are not strong. When a major case requires heavy recipes, the doctor must consider the physical conditions of the patient. If the patient is not strong enough to stand heavy recipes, drastic diaphoresis and purgatives may perish the *yang* and *yin* of the body. At any rate, one must be very careful in using heavy recipes.

8.2 SLOW-ACTING AND QUICK-ACTING RECIPES

Slow-acting recipe is composed of ingredients acting slowly

or counteracting each other to moderate effect and used in the treatment of chronic debilitated cases.

Typical is the Decoction of Four Nobles Ingredients, a basic slow-acting tonifying recipe for treating deficiency of vital energy of the spleen and stomach manifested by debility, lassitude, anorexia, etc. The recipe includes four ingredients: *renshen* (Radix Ginseng), *fuling* (Poria), *baizhu* (Rhizoma Atractylodis Macrocephalae), and *zhigancao* (Radix Glycyrrhizae Praeparata). The Black Plum Pills (*Wumei Wan*), a slow-acting recipe for treating chronic diarrhea, is composed of ten ingredients: *wumei* (black plum), *xixin* (Herba Asari), *ganjiang* (Dried Ginger), *zhifuzi* (Radix Aconiti Praeparata), *Guizhi* (Ramulus Cinnamomi), *renshen* (Radix Ginseng), *danggui* (Radix Angelicae Sinensis), *huanglian* (Rhizoma Coptidis), *huangbai* (Cortex Phellodendri), and *huajiao* (Pericarpium Zanthoxyli).

Quick-acting recipe is employed for immediate effect in the treatment of emergency or critical cases, such as cold limbs with sudden loss of consciousness up to above the knees and elbows, hardly felt pulse, etc.

The *Sini* Decoction is a quick-acting recipe. Consisting of *zhifuzi* (Radix Aconiti Praeparata), *ganjiang* (Dried Ginger) and *zhigancao* (Radix Glycyrrhizae Praeparata), it is used to restore vital function from collapse and shock with cold limbs.

Quick-acting recipes, usually with drastic drugs, are often accompanied by heavy recipes.

8.3 RECIPES WITH ONE OR MORE PRINCIPAL INGREDIENTS

The composition of recipes is decided by the cause of diseases. Recipes with one principal ingredient are used for treating diseases due to one simple cause. Recipes with more than two principal ingredients are for complicated diseases caused by many pathogenic factors. According to *The Internal Classic*, new diseases are usually simple and therefore one main ingredient is enough in a recipe; but prolonged illness often indicates complicated pathogenic factors and asks for recipes with more than two principal ingredients.

8.4 COMPOUND PRESCRIPTIONS

Compound prescriptions are formed by 1) many ingredients; 2) two or more set recipes.

Wuji Powder is a case in point. It is composed of four recipes: Decoction of Ephedra** (used as a diaphoretic and antasthmatic), Decoction of Cinnamon Twigs** (used to expel exogenous pathogenic factors from the exterior of the body and rectify derangement of the constructive and defensive systems), *Pingwei* Powder (consisting of atractytodes Rhixome, tangerine peel, magnolia bark and liguorice and is used for regulating the flow of vital energy and the function of the stomach), and *Erchen* Decoction** (which means Decoction of two old drugs: tangerine peel and pinllia tuber, and is used to resolve phlegm and regulate the function of the spleen and stomach).

With all these drugs put together, *Wuji* Powder functions differently from any of the original recipes. It is used mainly to subdue hyperactivity of the stomach, treating internal damage of vital energy as well as affection due to exogenous pathogenic factors.

In a word, to use compound prescriptions means to use several recipes at the same time to treat a special illness.

** For Decoction of Ephedra, Decoction of Cinnamon Twigs and Erchen Decoction, see Chapter 6 – 6.1, 6.2.

Chapter 9

Chinese Traditional Drugs

Chinese materia medica is an important component of Traditional Chinese medicine. Animals, plants, minerals can all be used as medicine, among which herbs are used most often.

The Tang Materia Medica (of the Seventh Century), China's first pharmacopoeia compiled by Su Jing and 22 other scholars, listed 844 medical substances. A more gigantic and comprehensive work, the world-famous *Compendium of Materia Medica*, was published in 1590. Compiled by Li Shizhen who worked 30 years on it, the 52-volume compendium listed 1,892 medical substances, and is still valued by pharmacists and botanists throughout the world. Li Shizhen's efforts were continued by Zhan Xuemin who wrote a supplement to the Compendium in 1765, in which 716 more medical substances were added.

Here are some basic ideas about Chinese traditional drugs.

9.1 FOUR PROPERTIES OF DRUGS

The four properties refer to cold, hot, warm and cool, classified according to their therapeutic effects.

Drugs effective for the treatment of heat symptom-complexes are endowed with cold or cool properties, while those effective for cold symptom-complexes, with warm or hot properties.

Evodia fruit and dried ginger, both endowed with warm or hot properties, are used for treating cold in the stomach manifested by stomach pain relieved by warmth, cold limbs and white coat of the tongue, etc.

There are of course drugs right in the middle. However, even those moderates may be with more or less cold and hot properties.

One of the important principles in Chinese medicine is that cold symptom-complex should be treated with drugs warm or hot in property, while heat symptom-complex should be treated with drugs cold in property. Drugs cold in property are used as antipyretics and febrifuges because they have the action to clear up internal heat. On the contrary, warming drugs like Radix Aconiti and Cortex Cinnamomi are used for dispelling internal cold, because they can restore *yang* (vital function) from collapse and warm up internal organs.

9.2 FIVE TASTES OF DRUGS

Referring to pungent, sweet, sour, bitter and salty, the tastes of drugs are different as are the properties. There are "tasteless" drugs, which are usually close to sweet.

Drugs sour in taste, such as schisandra fruit, Chinese gall, black plum, are used as astringents and hemostatics and can also treat seminal emission, night sweat, chronic diarrhea and prolapse of the anus.

Drugs pungent in taste can be used as diaphoretics and to regulate the flow of vital energy and blood and treat exterior symptom-complex caused by wind and cold. Representatives of pungent drugs are ephedra, cinammon twigs, cyperus tuber, etc.

Drugs sweet in taste can be used as tonics, mediator and in slow-acting prescriptions. There are drugs sweet in taste and cold in property such as scrophularia root, ophiopogon root, glehnia root, which can be used to nourish vital essence. There are also drugs sweet in taste but hot or warm in property, such as pilose Asiabell root and astraglus root, which can be used to strengthen vital energy.

Drugs bitter in taste, such as coptis root, phello-dendron bark and scutellaria root, are used to eliminate heat and dampness and stop diarrhea.

Drugs salty in taste can soften or clear stagnation of food or blood. Sargassum is used to treat scrofula; Exiccated Sodium Sulfate is good for treating constipation; and Oyster Shell can be used to soften and disperse hard lumps in the body.

Many drugs have mixed tastes, therefore with different functions.

9.3 COMBINATION OF DRUGS

Drugs are often put together with the purpose of producing desired therapeutic effect. But this must be done in a right way. Some drugs cannot go together and some can be applied only under given conditions.

The combination of more than two drugs must follow certain rules. China's earliest materia medica, *Shen Nong's Herbals*, which is believed to be a product of the first century B.C., recorded the following rules:

— Simple recipe: some single medical substances, such as ginseng, can treat an illness independently.

— Mutual reinforcement: two ingredients with similar properties are often used in combination to reinforce each other's action, e.g. Rhubarb and Mirabilite in the *Drastic Purgative Decoction.*

— Assistance: two or more ingredients in a prescription used in combination, one being the principal substance while the rest play a subsidiary role to reinforce the action of the former.

— Mutual restraint: the mutual restraining effect of different ingredients to weaken or neutralize each other's action, like pinellia tuber with fresh ginger.

— Neutralization: the property of one drug to neutralize the toxicity of another drug, like croton seed and mung bean.

— Incompatibility: the property of not being suitable for combination or simultaneous administration. Severe side effects may result when two incompatible ingredients are used in combination. Kansui root, for instance, must not be combined with Liquorice.

— Counteraction: the property of one drug to check the action of another drug, as asarum herb (Herba Asari) to Astraglus root (Radix Astragali).

As it is thus explained, those belonging to the categories of "mutual reinforcement" and "assistance" can be combined; and those falling in "mutual restraint", "counteraction" and "neutralization" should not go together; and those belonging to "incompatibility" must not be used simultaneously.

9.4 CONTRAINDICATIONS

Apart from rules guiding the combination of drugs, there are contraindications while taking Chinese drugs. Pregnant women should be especially cautious.

Different kinds of food should be abstained from while taking certain medicine: patients taking drugs with cold properties should avoid greasy food; patients taking drugs for warming up the lung and expelling phlegm should avoid raw and cold food; and those taking drugs for detumescence should avoid allergic food; etc.

Besides, meat should be abstained from while taking drugs like coptis root, platycodon root and black plum. Vinegar should be avoided while taking poria.

Generally speaking, cold, raw, sticky and greasy food

should all be avoided.

As for pregnant women, an ancient song listed more than 30 drugs that should not be taken, among which are dried ginger, pinellia tuber, ricepaper pith, pink (Herba Dianthi), croton seed, peach kernel, glayfly, leech, centipede, etc. According to the theory, pregnant women should especially abstain from drugs with drastic cold or hot properties and drastic drugs that apt to disintegrate stagnated vital energy and eradicate blood stasis.

Special attention should be paid to toxic drugs. When they are used together, their toxicity may become stronger. Sometimes, non-toxic drugs, when go together, can also produce serious side-effect. For instance, a man's circulation system may be blocked and breathing center paralyzed by taking ginseng and hellebore at the same time. Taking an overdose of the two may even lead to death.

Ancient Chinese summed up 18 incompatible medicaments which, if given in combination, are believed to give rise to serious side effects, and 19 medicaments of mutual restraint which, if used in combination, may restrain or neutralize each other's action. This is the advice offered by experienced people, and therefore merits keen attention.

The Eighteen Incompatible Medicaments are: *gancao* (Radix Glycyrrhizae) incompatible with *gansui* (Radix Euphorbiae Kansui), *jingdaji* (Radix Euphorbiae Pekinensis), *yuanhua* (Flos Genkwa), and *haizao* (Sargassum);

wutou (Radix Aconiti) incompatible with *beimu* (Bulbus Fritillariae), *gualou* (Fructus Trichosanthis), *banxia* (Rhizoma Pelliniae), *bailian* (Radix Ampelopsis), and *baiji* (Rhizoma Bletillae);

lilu (Radix Veratri Nigri) incompatible with *renshen* (Radix Ginseng), *shashen* (Radix Glehniae), *danshen* (Radix Salviae Miltiorrhizae), *kushen* (Radix Sophorae Flavescentis), *xixin* (Herba Asari) and *baishao* (Radix Paeoniae).

The Ninteen Medicaments of Mutual Restraint are:

liuhuang (sulfur) restraining *mangxiao* (crude mirabilite);

shuiyin (mercury) restraining *pishuang* (arsenic);

langdu (Radix Euphorbiae Ebracteolatae) restraining *mituoseng* (litharge);

badou (Semen Crotonis) restraining *qianniuzi* (Semen Pharbitidis);

dingxiang (Flos Caryophylli) restraining *yujin* (Radix Curcumae);

yaxiao (crystallized mirabilite) restraining *sanleng* (Rhizoma Sparganii);

chuanwu (Radix Aconiti) and *caowu* (Radix Aconiti Kusnezoffii) restraining *xijiao* (Cornu Rhinoceri);

renshen (Radix Ginseng) restraining *wulingzhi* (Paeces Trogopterorum);

rougui (Cortex Cinnamomi) restraining *chishizhi* (Halloysitum Rubrum).

Chapter 10

Common Diseases and Their Prevention and Cure

Common diseases include influenza, stomach trouble, chronic bronchitis, constipation, contraception, etc. Ways of prevention and recipes for the treatment of such diseases are introduced here.

10.1 TREATMENT OF INFLUENZA

Influenza usually has an incubation period of two or three days. Patients often have chills and fever, or a headache. They may have pain in the limbs, back and waist. They often have no appetite and feel tired. This disease is contagious. Patients may, at the same time, have tracheitis or inflammation in the throat and nasal cavity. In some cases, hidden measles may be found at the same time.

Commonly used recipe for influenza:
Lu gen 12g Bai mao gen 12g Sang zhi 15g
Sang ye 6g   Bo he 5g   Dan dou chi 9g
Chi shao 6g Jing jie 5g   Lian qiao 9g
Shan zhi 5g Dan zhu ye 5g

(To be taken after being simmered in water.)

10.1.1 Influenza with tracheitis

Symptoms: stuffed nose or running nose, tearful eyes, tonsils swollen, hoarse voice, high fever, coughing with or without phlegm, etc.

Treatment:

Prescription should be based on the commonly used recipe for influenza.

With coughing, add: Qian hu 5g Xing ren 5g;
With stuffed nose, add: Jie geng 5g Xin yi 5g;
With swelling pain in the brows, add:
   Ju hua 6g Bai zhi 3g;
With eyes hurt to light, add: Cao jue ming 9g;
With tinnitus, add: Chan tui yi 5g;
With swollen tonsils, add: Pu gong ying 9g
   Ban lan gen 9g Niu bang zi 5g;
With hoarse voice, add: Feng huang yi 5g
   Jin deng long 5g;
With headache, add: Man jing zi 5g;
With a tendancy to pneumonia, add: Ma huang 1g,
   Gui zhi 3g Shi gao 15g Ting li zi 3g;
With dizziness, add: Bai wei 6g;
With pain in the limbs and back, add:
   Gui zhi 3g Bai shao 9g Sang ye 15g.

10.1.2 Influenza with stomach trouble and intestine trouble

Treatment of this disease can be based on the commonly used recipe for influenza.

If the patient has a bad appetite, add:
   Pei lan ye 9g Xie bai 6g;
With a strnage odour in the mouth, add:
   Gua lou gen 6g
With thick and greasy coating of the tongue, add:
   Ji nei jin 9g Jiao san xian 15g;
With vomiting, add:
   Zhu ru 6g Ban xia 9g;
With dysentery, add: Bian dou yi 9g;

With pain in the stomach, add:
  Bai shao 9g   Xiang fu tan 6g;
With aching hernia (usually caused by constipation), add:
  Gua lou 15g

Note: the above dosage is for adults. For children the dosage should be reduced accordingly.

For patients who prefer taking prepared medicine like pills and medical granules, the following medicines are recommended when treating influenza.

a) *Gan mao qing re san chong ji* (medical granule to clear up internal heat and cure cold)

Ingredients:
  Jie sui, Bo he, Fang feng, Chai hu, Su ye, Xing ren,
  Jie geng, Zi hua di ding, Lu gen, Ge gen, Bai zhi
  (To be taken twice a day with the granule dissolved in boiling water.)

b) *Yin qiao jie du wan* (febrifugal pills of Lonicera and Forsythia)

Ingredients:
  Yin hua, Lian qiao, Jie geng, Niu bang zi, Bo he,
  Dan zhu ye, Jie sui, Dan dou chi, Gan cao

c) *Sang ju gan mao pian* (tablets of Mori and Chrysanthemum)

Ingredients:
  Sang ye, Ju hua, Lian qiao, Bo he, Xing ren, Jie geng,
  Lu geng, Gan cao

The above-mentioned prepared medicines are used as diaphoretic, febrifugal and detoxicant remedy for the treatment of early stage of influenza with headache, stuffed nose, sore throat, etc. Patients may take four to six tablets of *Sang ju gan mao pian* in the morning and one pill of *Yin qiao jie du wan* in the evening for three successive days, and be, in most cases, cured then.

d) *Ling qiao jie du wan/pian* (Febrifugal Pills/Tablets of Cornu Antelopis and Forsythia)

The pills consist of Cornu Antelopis and the ingredients of *Yin qiao jie du wan*. It is used to eliminate heat and dispel pathogenic factors from the exterior of the body by diaphoresis.

e) *Huo xiang zheng qi wan* (Pills for Dispelling Turbidity with Agastache)

This medicine is used for the treatment of influenza with stomach trouble and intestine trouble.

Ingredients:
Huo xiang, Hou po, Zi su ye, Jie geng, Chen pi,
Fu ling, Ban xia, Bai zhu, Bai zhi, Gan cao

f) *Jin yi qu shu wan* (Pills for Summer Diseases)

This medicine is used for the treatment of influenza with stomach trouble and intestine trouble.

Ingredients:
Fu ling, Huo xiang, Mu gua, Ding xiang, Zi su ye,
Xiang ru, Tan xiang

Huo xiang zheng qi wan and *Jin yi qu shu wan* are preferred in treating influenza in summer and autumn, when patients often suffer from sunstroke or cold, stomachache, vomiting and diarrhea. These pills are also used to treat acute gastroenteritis in summer and autumn.

When using diaphoretic method to treat exterior symptom-complex, attention should be paid to the treatment of interior symptom-complex. For instance, some one may have chilliness, headache, etc. in the exterior, and fever, heat in the stomach, food stagnancy, etc. in the interior at the same time. The recipes introduced above paid attention to both aspects. Take *Yin qiao jie du wan* for example. It contains drugs which can remove interior heat (Yin hua, Lian qiao, Niu bang zi, Jie geng) and drugs which can resolve interior heat (Bo he, Jie sui, Dan dou chi, Lu gen.)

It is very important for doctors to make an overall analysis of the patients' physical condition and distinguish the interior symptom-complex from the exterior symptom-complex before giving the prescription.

10.1.3 Example cases

Name of patient: Wang Aping　　Age: three
Symptoms: sore throat, high fever, headache, anorexia, constipation and darkish yellow urine, etc.
Prescription:
　　Lu gen　9g　　Bai mao gen　9g　　Dan dou chi　6g
　　Jin yin teng　5g　　Jin yin hua　5g　　Shuang gou teng　6g
　　Di long　5g　　Man jing zi　3g　　Chan tui yi　3g
　　Xing ren　5g　　Shan zhi　3g　　Fu ling　6g
　　Chi shao　6g　　Sang Ye　5g　　Sang zhi　9g
　　Ju hua　5g　　Jie geng　3g　　Chang pu　3g
　　Niu Bang zi　5g

The patient was fully recovered after taking two dosages of the medicine.

Explanatory note:

In this prescription, *Man jing zi, Dan dou chi,* and *Chan tui yi* are to resolve exterior symptoms, while *Lu gen, Bai mao ge,* and *Shan zhi* can relieve heat in the interior. *Chi shao* is used to eliminate evil heat from the blood, and *Gou teng* and *Di long* to ease the nerves and subdue convulsions. *Sang ye, Xing ren, Jie geng* are expectorants, and *Ju hua* has the function of relieving pain by dispelling wind and fever. Besides, *Jing yin hua* and *Jin yin teng* can cure the inflammation of the throat.

Name of patient: Wang Shen　Age: three
Symptoms: had stuffed food, and then caught cold, also had tracheitis, a little fever, vomited some mucus sometimes, etc.

Prescription:
   Qian hu 3g   Bai qian 3g   Zi yuan 5g
   Chi shao 5g   Xing ren 5g   Jie geng 3g
   Pei lan ye 6g   Lu gen 6g   Bai mao gen 6g
   Lai fu zi 5g   Lai fu ying 5g   Sang bai pi 3g
   Sang ye 5g   Jiao san xian 9g   Zhi qiao 3g
   Gan cao 1.5g   Zi su zi 3g   Fu ling 5g
         (two dosages)

Explanatory note:
   Lu gen and *Bai mao gen* are antipyretics. They help resolve exterior fever. *Fu ling* and *Chi shao* help resolve interior fever. *Qian hu, Bai qian, Zi yuan, Zi su zi, Xing ren, Sang bai pi* and *Sang ye* are all good cough remedies. *Xing ren*, when ground, is good laxative. The patient vomits because of indigestion. *Jiao san xian* and *Zhi qiao* can help promote digestion and remove food stagnancy. To relieve distention and dispel phlegm, *Lai fu zi* and *Lai fu ying* are used.
   The patient was recovered after taking the medicine.

10.2 TREATMENT OF STOMACH TROUBLE

A recipe is recommended for stomach trouble with the following symptoms: cold in the stomach, constant stomachache, nauseating, vomiting (watery fluid), etc.
Ingredients:
   Rou gui 6g   Gao liang jiang 6g   Bi bo 6g
   Mu xiang 6g   Ji nei jin 9g   Fu shou 9g
      (Grind the drugs add 200g Sodium bicarbonate and mix them well. Take one spoonful of the powder each time, twice a day, once in the morning, once in the evening.)

Explanatory note:
   This medicine is effective for curing chronic gastritis. *Rou gui, Gao liang jiang, Bi bo* and *Mu xiang* are drugs for

dispelling internal cold by warming up the stomach. They are used for the treatment of cold and pain in the stomach. *Ji nei jin* and *Fu shou* are carminative and stomachic. They can produce a better effect when used with sodium bicarbonate, which can help with digestion.

10.3 TREATMENT OF NAUSEA AND VOMITING DURING EARLY PREGNANCY

The most troublesome women diseases are dysmenorrhea and morning sickness (nausea and vomiting during early pregnancy.) Morning sickness usually starts in the second month of pregnancy. Patients nauseate or vomit after eating. They may favour sour and hot things, or drool for things like children. They get tired of food they used to like. Sometimes they feel very tired, dizzy, hot and have no appetite.

This perios may last for three months or even throughout the whole pregnancy period.

Here are two example prescriptions.

I.
Bian dou 30g   Wu zhu yu 0.6g   Huang lian 2.4g
Ji li 9g   Hou po 5g   Mei gui hua 5g
Sha ren 5g   Bai dou kou 5g   Xuan fu hua 6g
Ban xia 6g   Zi su ye 3g   Huang qin 9g
Zhi qiao 5g   Bai zhu 5g   Chen pi 6g   Zhu ru 6g
   (Boil and simmer the drugs in water. Take half of the decoction in the morning, the other half in the evening. Three dosages to be taken in three days.)

II.
Sha ren 5g   Bai Dou kou 5g   Xuan fu hua 6g
Ban xia 9g   Hou po 5g   Mei kui hua 5g
Yue ji hua 5g   Bian dou 10g   Chen pi 6g
Huang qin 9g   Bai zhu 6g   Zhu ru 6g
Pei lan ye 9g   Wu zhu yu 1.5g   Huang lian 1.5g
Dao ya 15g   Xie bai 6g   Xi yang shen 3g

(Three dosages)

Explanatory notes:
Chen pi, Bian dou are stomachic, Sha ren, Bai dou kou, Zi su ye are used as stomach-warming agent for the treatment of nausea, vomiting, Wu Zhu yu and Huang lian are used to eliminate heat in the liver, Bai zhu is used to invigorate the function of the spleen and stomach and together with Huang qin can be used for the treatment of hypertension and threatened abortion. Xi yang shen is used to replenish vital essence. Mei gui hua, Yue ji hua, Pei lan are drugs with fragrant odour for resolving dampness and for the treatment of poor appetite.

These two prescriptions have been proved to be effective in clinic practice.

10.4 TREATMENT OF TRACHEITIS CAUSED BY COLD

Prescription:
   Feng huang yi 7g   Jie geng 6g   He zi 6g
   Xing ren 6g   Fu ling 12g   Huang qin 9g
   Sang ye 15g   Qian hu 6g   Zi su zi 6g
   Zi yuan 9g   Ju hong 6g   Gua lou 9g
   Tian hua fen 12g   Dai ge san 6g   Pi pa ye 9g
   Gan cao 3g   Five Dates
   (Three dosages were needed, taken in three days.)

Explanatory notes:
This medicine is used to treat cold with coughing, sore throat, and tracheitis. Feng huang yi, Jie geng, He zi are used to treat hoarse and sore throat; Zi su zi, Qian hu, Ju hong are used to treat coughing and resolve phlegm; Sang zhi, Sang ye, to dispell evil wind and cure pain; Pi pa ye is used as antitussive, expectorant; Dates are cardiac stimulant.

10.5 RECIPE FOR CHRONIC BRONCHITIS

Some old people suffer from chronic bronchitis. When the weather turns cold, they would suffer from coughing, profuse phlegm and asthma. It is advisable to make some soft extract according to the following prescription, and take it regularly, which is convenient and effective.

Prescription:
    Xian ren dou 2 pieces   Bei mu 60g   Bai mao gen 150g
    Walnut kernel 120g   7 White Pears (with seeds removed)
    Tea 30g   7 Chinese Dates

    Put all these ingredients into a pot, add water and simmer them until mashed. Filtrate and concentrate the decoction, add 60g honey, go on simmering till it turns to a syrup.

    Store the syrup in a porcelain container. Take one spoonful of it each time, three times a day.

10.6 RECIPE FOR THREATENED ABORTION

Prescription:
    Lao zong tan 30g   Di yu 9g   E jiao 9g
    Gui ban 9g   Sheng di 9g   Shu di huang 9g
    Ai ye 6g   Dang gui 15g   Rice Vinegar 60g
    (Two dosages)

Note:
This prescription was very effective in use. Bleeding stopped with only two dosages of medicine.

Lao zong tan and Di yu are used as astringent hemostatics and anti-diarrheal with the effect of eliminating evil heat from the blood for the treatment of bleeding. E jiao and Gui ban are used to nourish the blood and to stop bleeding. Dang gui is blood tonic. Rice vinegar, sour and puckery, can help other drugs enhance their actions.

10.7 RECIPE FOR BED-WETTING

Prescription:
    Bai guo 7 pieces   Sang piao xiao 9g   Wu yao 9g
       Taken twice a day for five days, (simmered in water) then once every other day until cured.

Note:
This dosage is for children under five years old. For those older, dosage should be increased to:
    Bai guo 14 pieces   Sang piao xiao 15g   Wu yao 15g
(Bai guo beaten with shells, then simmered in water with the other ingredients.)

10.8 TREATMENT OF INFANT CONSTIPATION

Prescription:
    Shan zha 9g   Bing lang 9g   Shen qu 9g
    Mai ya 9g
       (The patient was cured after taking the medicine once.)

10.9 TREATMENT OF INSOMNIA

Prescription:
    Suan zao ren 15g   Long yan rou 15g   Wu wei zi 9g
       (Simmered in water, and taken once in the morning, once in the evening)

10.10 RECIPE FOR CONTRACEPTION

Prescription:
    Ku ding cha 15g   Gong lao ye 15g
       (To be taken for three successive days after each menstruation.)

10.11 TREATMENT OF OLD PEOPLE'S CONSTIPATION

Old people's constipation is often caused by peristaltic difficulty or insufficiency of blood in the small intestine.
Prescription:
  Rou cong rong 60g   Bei sha shen 30g   Xing ren 6g
  Zi wan 6g   Dang gui 30g

> (Put all these ingredients into a pot, add water and simmer them till mashed. Filtrate and concentrate the decoction, add honey, and go on simmering till it turns to a syrup. Take a spoonful of it each time, once in the morning once in the evening.)

10.12 TREATMENT OF CORONARY HEART DISEASE

Prescription: (I)
  Chi shao 15g   Chuan xiong 15g   Hong hua 15g
  Ji xue teng 30g   Dan shen 3g   San leng 18g
  Yuan hu 15g   Jiang xiang 15g   Xie bai 18g
  Ji xing zi 12g

Prescription (II):
  Shan zha 24g   Huang jing 15g   Kun bu 15g
  Yuan hu 6g   Bai zi ren 9g   Chang pu 9g
  Yu jin 9g

Prescription (III):
  Di jin cao 9g   Xian he cao 12g   Long yan rou 12g
  Bai zi ren 9g   Yuan zhi 6g   Mai dong 9g
  Wu wei zi 6g   Tai zi shen 12g

10.13 TONICS FOR OLD PEOPLE

This medicine can help old people replenish vital energy,

and give the body more strength.

Ingredients:

 Huang qi 240g Shu di huang 240g Huang jing 240g
 Hei zhi ma 120g Hei dou 240g Fu ling 240g
 Qian shi 240g Long gu 60g Zi he che 60g
 Yuan shen 60g Mai dong 30g Shan yao 240g
 Ce bai ye 120g Hu po 15g

> (These drugs should be powdered first, and then mixed and made into small globular mass with honey as excipient called "honeyed bolus", each weighing 9g.
> Take one bolus each time, once in the morning, once in the evening.)

10.14 BLOOD TONICS — for Nourishing the Blood and Regulating Blood Conditions

Ingredients:

 Yi mu cao 240g Ji xue teng 240g Yi mu cao zi 90g
 Yue ji hua 90g Dang gui 90g Qian cao 60g
 Chuan xiong 30g Bai shao 60g Chi shao 60g
 Sheng di huang 60g Shu di huang 60g
 Chai hu 30g Dan shen 120g Dan pi 60g
 Ze lan 60g Hong hua 60g Tao ren 90g
 Jie geng 45g Xiang fu 90g Zi su geng 45g
 Zhi qiao 60g Yuan hu 60g Qiang huo 15g
 E jiao 120g Chuan shan jia 90g Ai ye 30g
 Bie jia 90g Chuan lian zi 60g Gan cao 60g
 Ju he 60g Li zhi he 60g

> (These drugs should be powdered, then mixed; Add honey and make into boluses, each weighing 9 g. To be taken with warm boiled water. One bolus in the morning, one in the evening.)

This medicine is used for gynecological diseases such as menstrual disorders, advanced or retarded menstruation, dysmenorrhea, irregular menstruation, etc. It should not be taken by pregnant women.

10.15 TEN RECIPES OF DR. SHI JINMO

10.15.1 Recipe for the treatment of cirrhosis of the liver

Prescription:

Chai hu 45g   Bai shao 60g   Yu jin 30g
Rou gui 15g   Bai zhu 60g   E zhu 30g   San leng 30g
Chuan xiong 30g   Chuan lian zi 30g   Hou po 30g
Zhi shi 60g   Chen pi 15g   Dang gui 30g
Qian niu zi 30g   Guang mu xiang 15g   Hu po 30g
Cang zhu 30g   Sha ren 15g   Bing lang 30g
Qing pi 15g   Fu ling 60g   Ren shen 30g
Tao ren 30g   Xue jie 30g   Dan pi 30g   Ban xia 30g
Wu yao 30g   Gan cao 30g   Di long 30g

(These ingredients be powdered and mixed, then with water and flour paste as excipient, made into small globular mass or "watered pills". Each time take 5g of the pills, once in the morning, once in the evening, with warm boiled water.)

10.15.2 Recipe for oedematous liver or spleen

Prescription:

Bie jia 60g   Bai zhu 30g   Yuan hu 30g
Qian cao 30g   Chai hu 30g   E zhu 30g
Ru xiang 30g   Dang gui 30g   Xiang fu 30g
Chi shao 30g   Bai shao 30g   Dan pi 30g
San leng 30g   Wu yao 30g   Ji nei jin 30g
Ma bian cao 30g   Chi xiao dou 60g   Gui ban 60g
Cang zhu 30g   Hua shi 60g   She xiang 6g
Wu ling zhi 30g   Wa leng zi 60g   Long dan cao 24g
San qi 30g   Xue yu tan 30g   Bai jiang cao 60g
Gan cao 30g

(Be powdered, mixed and made into pills. Take 5 – 6 g of the pills each time, once in the morning, once in the evening with warm boiled water.)

10.15.3 Recipe for the treatment of gastric ulcer

Prescription:
  Gan cao 120g   Bo he 30g   Hai piao xiao 60g
  Shi chang pu 30g   Shen qu 60g   Bai zhu 60g
  Mu xiang 15g   Zhi shi 30g   Wu yao 30g
  Ji nei jin 60g   Sha ren 15g   Chen pi 15g
  Mo yao 30g   Ru xiang 30g   Fu ling 60g
  Dang gui 30g   Dan pi 60g   San qi 30g
  Tan xiang 15g   Bai shao 30g

  (To be powdered and mixed. Take 3g of the powder each time, once in the morning, once in the evening. This medicine can be taken for three successive months.)

10.15.4 Recipe for the treatment of duodenal ulcer

Prescription:
  Ku shen 60g   Chai hu 30g   Bai jiang cao 60g
  Xian he cao 60g   Hua shi 60g   Huang lian 30g
  Cang zhu 30g   Bai zhu 30g   Ci wei pi 60g
  Xiang fu mi 60g   Dan pi 30g   E jiao 60g
  Zhi qiao 60g   Yuan hu 30g   Qing pi 15g
  Chen pi 15g   Hou po 30g   Chi shao 30g
  Bai shao 30g   Bi bo 15g   Gan cao 30g
  Feng wei cao 30g

  (To be made into boluses with honey as excipient, each weighing 9g. Take one bolus each time, once in the morning, once in the evening.)

10.15.5 Recipe for the treatment of chronic dysentery

Prescription:
  Hei dou 90g   Shi lian rou 60g   Qian shi 60 g
  Huang lian 60g   Chun gen pi 60g   Jin ying zi 60g
  Mu xiang 30g   Bai shao 60g   Dang gui 30g
  Di yu 30g   Zhi qiao 30g   Ji cai 60g

Jin yin hua 90g   Ku shen 60g   Lao zong tan 60g
Dang shen 60g   Gan cao 120g

(To be powdered and mixed, and made into pills with rice vinegar as excipient. Take 6g of the pills each time, once before breakfast, once in the evening.)

10.15.6   Recipe for chronic enteritis

Prescription:

Pu er cha 60g   Gan jiang 30g   He zi 30g
Mi qiao 45g   Fu ling 60g   Hong ren shen 30g
Bai zhu 60g   Fu zi 30g   Wu wei zi 30g
Bu gu zhi 30g   Liu huang 30g   Chang zhu 30g
Rou dou kou 30g   Wu zhu yu 15g   Chen pi 15g
Ban xia 30g   Huang lian 30g   Gan cao 30g

(Powdered and mixed, then made into small pills with *Shen qu* and water as excipient.

Take 6g of the pills every morning and evening.)

10.15.7   Recipe for the treatment of cirrhosis with ascites

Prescription:

Bi cheng qie 30g   Fu zi 30g   Yuan hua 30g
Jing da ji 30g   Fu ling 60g   Rou gui 15g
Shang lu 30g   Gui zhi 30g   Chen xiang 12g
Mu xiang 15g   Ze xie 30g   Cao dou kou 12g
Bai zhu 60g   She xiang 6g   Zhu ling 30g
Hong hua zi 30g   Tao ren 30g

(Powdered and mixed, then made into pills with vinegar as excipient and *Hua shi* as coating. Take 3-4g of the pills every morning and evening with warm boiled water.)

10.15.8   Recipe for the treatment of cirrhosis with jaundice

Prescription:

Yu jin 60g   Bie jia 60g   Yin chen 60g

Hu po 30g Zi he che 60g Huang lian 30g
Chi shao 30g Bai shao 30g Shen qu 30g
Ku fan 15g Hong hua 30g Sheng di huang 60g
Mang xiao 15g Dang gui 30g Zhi shi 30g
Chai hu 30g Huang qi 60g Xiong dan 15g
Gan cao 15g

(To be powdered and mixed and made into pills. Take 6g of the pills once in the morning, once in the evening with warm boiled water.)

10.15.9 Recipe for the treatment of cholelith and jaundice

Prescription:
Ku fan 15g Mang xiao 15g Hua shi 60g
Yu zhen gu 45g Yu jin 60g Xiong dan 15g
E zhu 30g Yin chen 60g Xiang fu mi 60g
Shan zhi 30g Da huang 15g Huang qin 30g
Huang lian 15g

(To be made into pills after being powdered and mixed. Take 2g of the pills every morning and evening.)

10.15.10 Recipe for the treatment of dilatation and ptosis of the stomach

Prescription:
Bai zhu 60g Zhi shi 60g Sheng ma 15g
Chai hu 15g He zi 15g Ku geng 30g
Rou gui 15g Xi xin 15g Ren shen 30g
Huang lian 15g Gao liang jiang 15g
Chen pi 15g Wu zhu yu 15g Xie bai 15g
Dang gui 15g Chuan xiong 15g Gan cao 30g
Sha ren 15g Yuan hu 15g Cang zhu 30g
Wu yao 15g Min jiang 15g Huo xiang 15g
Chang pu 15g

(To be powdered and mixed. Take 3g of the mixed powder every morning and evening.)

These ten recipes were proved to be effective in Shi Jinmo's long years' clinical practice.

For the introduction to Shi Jinmo, see Chapter 11.

Chapter 11

Records of Shi Jinmo's Clinical Practice

Shi Jinmo (1881-1969) was a native of Zhejian Province, southeast China, but his footmarks had been left in many parts of the country, as an educator and foremost as a renowned practioner of Chinese medicine.

His career as a doctor started when he was only 13 years old and studying medicine with his uncle, a well-known doctor in a central China province. He later entered a law school and once served as a provincial minister of education at the early years after the 1911 Revolution. But his increasing reputation in medicine and perhaps also weariness of politics made him finally engaged in the research and practice of Chinese medicine, a career to which he devoted the rest of his life until his death at the age of 88.

After 1949, Shi served as vice-president of Chinese Medical Society, vice-chairman of the academy committee of the Academy of Traditional Chinese Medicine and advisor to several major hospitals in Beijing.

An advocate of combining traditional Chinese medicine with Western medicine, he was among the few people who first introduced western terminology to traditional Chinese medicine. He also named a number of his patent medicines with modern terms.

Shi was especially good at combining various ingredients in a prescription with the purpose of producing desired therapeutic effect in unison and reducing toxic or side effects. He often used two drugs simultaneously to produce opposite effects: both cold and warm, or treating interior and exterior symptoms, etc. People called them "Shi's Matching Drugs."

11.1 TREATMENT OF STOMACH TROUBLE

Stomach trouble is a common disease, which is often caused by over-eating or indigestion, etc. Patients often have the following symptoms: stomachache, nausea, belching, hiccuping, vomiting, etc. They usually have a thick coating on the tongue and a bad smell in the mouth.

11.1.1 Example case 1
Name of patient: Zhang
Symptoms: suffering from chronic gastritis and indigestion, having excessive acidity, etc.
Treatment:
First prescription:
Xuan fu hua 6g   Zhe shi 9g   Xiang fu mi 9g
Dao ya 15g   Dan shen 9g   Wu zhu yu 0.6g
Huang lian 3g   Chen pi tan 6g   Ji nei jin 9g
Pei lan ye 9g   Jie geng 5g   Su geng 5g
Zhi qiao 5g   Gan jiang tan 0.9g

After taking two dosages of this medicine, the patient felt better. But he still had that thick coating on the tongue, an uneasy feeling in his stomach, and suffering from constipation.

Second prescription:
Gua lou 12g   Xuan fu hua 6g   Jiang zhong po 5g
Xie bai 6g   Zhe shi 9g   Chen pi tan 6g

Ji nei jin 9g   Pei lan ye 9g   Mang xiao 3g
Zhi qiao 5g   Tao ren 6g   Xing ren 6g
Lai fu zi 5g   Lai fu ying 5g   Ban xia 10g
Zuo jin wan 6g

After taking two dosages of this medicine, the patient felt even better, though he sometimes still felt pain in the stomach, and his appetite was not normal yet.

Third prescription:
Hou po hua 5g   Dai dai hua 5g   Xi yang shen 5g
Tao ren 6g   Xing ren 6g   Dan shen 12g
Gua lou 12g   Xie bai 6g   Shen qu 9g
Pei lan ye 9g   Ji nei jin 9g   Mei gui hua 5g
Gu ya 9g   Mai ya 9g   Zhi qiao 5g   Gan cao 6g

The patient was recovered after taking three dosages of the third prescription, and regained his appetite. In order to consolidate the effect, the doctor suggested he take patent pills for ten more days.

Prescription:
In the morning, take *Xiang sha yang wei wan* 6g
In the evening, take *Bao he wan*, one pill
   (To be taken with warm boiled water)

11.1.2 Example case 2
Name of patient: Zhao   Age: 35
Symptoms: Often felt painful and stuffed in the stomach, belching, stools dry and hard, etc.
Treatment:
First prescription:
Gua lou 24g   Xie bai 9g   Bai zhi ma 30g
Xuan fu hua 6g   Zhe shi 12g   Shi di 9g
Hou po 5g   Ding xiang 0.6g   Chen pi tan 6g
Ji nei jin 9g   Shen qu 6g   Zhi qiao 5g
Bai zhu 5g   Sha ren 3g   Bai dou kou ren 3g
Dan shen 15g   Huai niu xi 9g

The patient felt a little better after taking three dosages of the medicine, but still suffered from constipation.

Second prescription:
Can sha 9g   Zao jiao zi 9g   Lai fu zi 6g
Lai fu ying 6g   Gua lou 18g   Bai zhi ma 30g
Chen pi tan 6g   Niu xi 9g   Hou po 5g
Gong ding xiang 5g   Shi di 6g   Xuan fu hua 6g
Zhe shi 9g   Sha ren 5g   Bai dou kou ren 5g
Xing ren 6g   Ban xia 6g   Bai zhu 5g
Zhi qiao 5g

The patient was fully recovered after taking three dosages of this medicine.

11.1.3 Example case 3
Name of patient: Liu   Age: 30
Symptoms: Having suffered from gastric ulcer for more than a year; often had stomachache, vomited often, had occult blood in the stool.
Treatment:
First prescription:
Chi shao 6g   Bai shao 6g   Ru xiang 5g
Mo yao 5g   Pu gong ying 9g   Chai hu 5g
Tao ren 6g   Xing ren 6g   Dan zhu ye 6g
Gua lou 15g   Xie bai 9g   Wu zhu yu 0.6g
Huang lian 3g   Yuan ming fen 6g   Zhu ru 6g
Jin yin hua 12g   Gan cao 3g

The patient vomited less often, the pain relieved a little, after taking two dosages. He went to see the doctor again.

Second prescription:
Xuan fu hua 6g   Zhe shi 9g   Xue yu tan 9g
Zuo jin wan 6g   Dan shen 12g   Dan pi 6g
Jin yin teng 12g   Pu gong ying 9g   Lao jun tan 5g
Ru xiang 4.5g   Mo yao 4.5g   Zhu ru 6g

Chi shao 6g   Bai shao 6g   Chai hu 5g
  (two dosages, taken on two successive days)

Third prescription:
Xuan fu hua 6g   Zhe shi 15g   Hou po 5g
Dai dai hua 5g   Dan shen 12g   Dan pi 6g
Pu gong ying 9g   Bai jiang cao 9g   Ci gu 9g
Gua lou 15g   Mang xiao 5g   Xue yu tan 9g
Ban xia 6g   Shen qu 6g   Wu zhu yu 0.6g
Huang lian 3g   Gan cao 5g
  (three dosages)

Fourth prescription:
Ci gu 9g   Bai jiang cao 9g   Bai shao 9g
Xuan fu hua 6g   Zhe shi 15g   Hou po 5g
Mei gui hua 5g   Dan pi 6g   Dan shen 15g
Sha ren 5g   Bai dou kou 5g   Tao ren 6g
Xing ren 6g   Zuo jin wan 6g   Xue yu tan 9g
Pu gong ying 9g   E jiao 12g
  (three dosages)

After taking medicine according to the third and fourth prescriptions, the patient got much better. Stomachache was eased, and vomiting was stopped. But there was still some occult blood.

The doctor told him to take three more dosages of the fourth prescription, but added:
E jiao 12g   Xi yang shen 3g.
The patient regained his appetite.

Sixth prescription:
Long gu 15g   Mu li 15g   E jiao 12g
Bai shao 9g   Xue yu tan 9g   Zuo jin wan 6g
Hou po hua 5g   Mei gui hua 5g   Xi yang shen 3g
Bai jiang cao 9g   Sha shen 9g   Ji nei jin 9g
Gu ya 9g   Mai ya 9g

(four dosages)

The patient was fully recovered after taking the medicine.

11.2 TREATMENT OF HYPERTENSION

Hypertension refers to abnormally high blood pressure in the arteries, which is often accompanied by nervousness, dizziness and headaches. Traditional Chinese medicine believes that hypertension is caused by imbalance of *Yin* and *Yang*. It is often seen at the first stage to be exuberant in *Yang*, and then turns deficient in *Yin*. In the end, the patient may be deficient both in *Yin* and *Yang*. This disease should be treated by looking into both its root cause and its symptoms or complications.

11.2.1 Example case 1
Name of patient: Huang   Age: 61   Sex: female
Symptoms: Having suffered from hypertension for years, often felt dizzy, often had tinnitus and vomited, had pain in the waist, frequent urination, etc.
Treatment:
  First prescription:
  Ci shi 30g   Shi jue ming 30g   Xuan fu hua 6g
  Zhe shi 15g   Bai guo 10 pieces   Niu xi 15g
  Yuan zhi 9g   Bai wei 6g   Sha ji li 9g
  Ji li 9g   Fu shen 9g   Mai dong 9g
  Chan tui yi 5g   Ju hua 9g   Xia ku cao 9g
  Tian ma 5g   Du zhong 30g   Chang pu 6g
     (four dosages)

The patient felt better after taking the decoctions, but preferred to take pills.

  Second prescription:
  Ji li 60g   Mai dong 30g   Niu xi 30g

Shi jue ming 30g Wu zhu yu 15g Chuan xiong 15g
Fu shen 30g Sha ji li 30g Chang pu 30g
Yuan zhi 30g Nü zhen zi 30g Han lian cao 30g
Long dan cao 15g Chan tui yi 15g Ju hua 30g
Sang ye 30g Suan zao ren 30g Bai zi ren 30g
Sheng di 30g Shu di huang 30g Gou ji 30g
Du zhong 60g Sha ren 15g Gan cao 15g
(Powder and mix these ingredients, add honey as excipient and make them into pills, each weighing 9g. Take one pill every morning and one in the evening with warm boiled water.)

The patient was fully recovered after taking the medicine.

11.2.2 Example case 2

Name of patient: Han   Age: 32   Sex: male
Symptoms: high blood pressure, dizziness, palpitation and short of breath, dreamfulness, dyspepsia, etc.
Prescription:
Long chi 30g Shi jue ming 30g Ji li 30g
Dang shen 30g Niu xi 30g Yuan zhi 30g
Bai zi ren 30g Xuan fu hua 30g Fu shen 30g
Han lian cao 30g Suan zao ren 30g Gan cao 30g
Gou teng 30g Bai zhu 30g Lu jiao jiao 30g
Long dan cao 15g Du zhong 60g Bai wei 30g
Shen qu 30g Sha ren 15g
(To be made into pills with honey as excipient, each weighing 3g. Take one pill every morning and evening with warm boiled water.)

Explanation:

Among these drugs, some can help lower blood pressure. They are Du zhong, Niu xi, Shi jue ming, Xuan fu hua, Long dan cao, and Ji li. Some are sedatives and tranquilizers: Dang shen, Bai zi ren, Suan zao ren, Fu shen. Lu jiao jiao, Long chi, and Gou teng are drugs for reinforcing the vital function and nourishing the blood. Shen qu and Sha ren are digestives. These drugs cover up not only the root cause of the disease, but also its overall complications. The patient was recovered after taking the medicine.

11.3 TREATMENT OF NEURASTHENIA

Neurasthenia is a kind of neurosis, and a common disease, which is due to emotional conflict. As it is caused by functional disorder of the nervous system, it may be reflected in many internal organs. It is often seen with the following symptoms: dizziness, headache, insomnia, amnesia, palpitation, excessive fatigue, stuffed feeling in the chest, indigestion, etc.

In treating neurasthenia, the doctor should first analyse the symptoms and signs of the illness, including the cause, nature and location of it and the patient's physical condition and then use accordingly the following methods: check hyperactivity of the liver and soothe the nerves; subdue the hyperactivity of the liver and dispell pathogenic heat from the heart; soothe the liver and invigorate the function of the spleen; replenish vital essence of the liver; and tonify the kidney and nourish the liver.

11.3.1 Example case 1
Name of patient: Wang   Age: 35   Sex: male
Symptoms: often had headache and dizziness, tinnitus, forgetfullness, restless and dreamfulness in sleep, indigestion, etc.
First Prescription:
  Zi shi ying 9g   Zi bei chi 9g   Xuan fu hua 6g
  Zhe shi 9g   Fu shen 9g   Mai dong 6g
  Ji li 12g   Yuan zhi 9g   Chang pu 6g
  Hou po 6g   Mei gui hua 6g   Shi jue ming 18g
  Cao jue ming 9g   Gua lou 18g   Xie bai 9g
  Suan zao ren 12g   Ju hua 9g   Sang ye 6g
  Sang zhi 18g

After taking six dosages of the medicine, the patient felt better with his stomach trouble; the headache and dizziness stopped.

Second prescription:
   Take 30 pills of *Shen jing shuai ruo wan* in the morning.
   Take one pill of *Zhu sha an shen wan* in the evening.

The patient was recovered after taking pills according to the prescription for one month.

11.3.2 Example case 2
Name of patient: Zhang   Sex: male
Symptoms: suffering from neurasthenia, could not sleep well, often felt tired, dizzy and had headache, etc.
Prescription:
   Ji li 30g   Long chi 30g   Mu li 30g
   Yuan zhi 30g   Shi hu 30g   Fu shen 30g
   Mai dong 30g   Bai zi ren 30g   Shou wu teng 30g
   Lu jiao jiao 30g   Suan zao ren 30g   Bai wei 15g
   Gan cao 15g
   (Powder these drugs and mix them, then make the powder into pills using honey as excipient. Take 9g of the pills each time, once in the morning, once in the evening with warm boiled water.)

This medicine is good at nourishing the blood, soothing the nerves and invigorating the function of the heart. The patient was recovered after taking this medicine for three months.

11.3.3   Example case 3
Name of patient: Li   Age: 64   Sex: female
Symptoms: neurasthenia, and sometimes even mental disorder, restlessness, palpitation, dizziness and insomnia, etc.
Prescription:
   Bai he 12g   Sheng di huang 9g   Zhi mu 6g

E jiao 9g   Chang pu 6g   Bai wei 6g
Fu xiao mai 24g   Ji li 15g   Gan cao 6g
Long gu 9g   Mu li 9g   Dates (5 pieces)

The patient was recovered after taking five dosages of the decoction.

11.4   TREATING OF MIGRAINE

Headache is a symptom of neurasthenia. The treatment of migraine usually depends on which part of the head (the right or the left) aches. That's why the treatment of migraine is singled out from the treatment of neurasthenia.

11.4.1   Example case 1
Name of patient: Zhang Hairong   Age: 45   Sex: male
Symptoms: suffering from chronic neuritis, and often had aches on the left side of the head and left temple.
Prescription:
Man jing zi 6g   Long dan cao 5g   Bai jiang can 5g
Long gu 9g   Mu li 9g   Sheng di huang 9g
Shu di huang 9g   Sha ren 3g   Xi xin 3g
Chuan xiong 5g   Ji li 12g   Jie geng 5g
Gao ben 5g   Cang er zi 6g   Gan song 5g
Ju hua 9g   Sang ye 6g

The patient was recovered after taking three dosages of the medicine.

11.4.2   Example case 2
Name of patient: Xu   Age: 40   Sex: female
Symptoms: often had aching at the back of the head, also tinnitus and dreamfulness; pain increased during menstruation period; had phlegm in the morning, etc.

Prescription:
   Long gu 12g   Mu li 12g   Shi jue ming 18g
   Cao jue ming 9g   Ju hong 4.5g   Ju luo 4.5g
   Man jing zi 6g   Ji li 9g   Sha ji li 9g
   Hei zhi ma 30g   Zao ren 18g   Chan tui yi 4.5g
   Chuan xiong 4.5g   Ju hua 9g   Bai zhi 4.5g
   Sang ye 6g   Hou po hua 4.5g   Mei gui hua 4.5g
     (four dosages)

The patient felt well again after taking the medicine. But when menstruation period came, the aching returned. So she came to see the doctor for the second time.

Prescription:
   Long gu 12g   Mu li 12g   Ci zhu wan 6g
   Shu mi 12g   Sha ji li 9g   Ji li 9g
   Shou wu 9g   Lu jiao jiao 9g   Dang gui 9g
   Chuan xiong 4.5g   Huang qi 18g   Sheng di huang 6g
   Shu di huang 6g   Chai hu 4.5g   Hou po hua 6g
   Mei gui hua 6g   Wu zhu yu 4.5g   Huang lian 4.5g
   Sha ren 3g   Xi xin 3g   Bai shao 9g
   Bai zhi 4.5g   Gan cao 4.5g   Ban xia 9g
     (five dosages)

The patient was recovered after taking the medicine.

11.4.3   A brief introduction to the properties of the drugs generally used in treating migraine

Long gu, Mu li, Zi shi ying, Zi bei chi, Suan zao ren, Yuan zhi, Shou wu teng and *Hu po* all belong to the category of sedatives and tranquilizers. They are used for the treatment of palpitation, insomnia, dreamfulness, dizziness and convulsion due to neurasthenia and hypertension.

Wu wei zi is used as tonic for neurasthenia.

Shi hu can replenish the vital essence of the lung and spleen, clear up the excessive heat and promote the secretion of body fluids.

Gua lou and *Tian hua fen* are used for resolving phlegm

and relieving thirst.

Chuan xiong is used to invigorate blood circulation and promote the flow of vital energy, and relieve pain of the head.

Ju hong and *Ju luo* are antitussives.

Dang gui is a drug for nourishing the blood; and *Lu jiao jiao* is for reinforcing the vital function.

Shi jue ming, Cao jue ming, Ji li and *Sha ji li* are anti-convulsives, which are used to subdue the hyperactivity of the liver and dispel the wind and clear the eyes.

Bai zhi can dispel the wind and invigorate blood. It is very effective in treating headaches.

Chan tui yi is used to treat tinnitus.

Hou po hua and *Mei gui hua* can cure the pain in the stomach and improve digestion.

11.5 TREATMENT OF DIABETES

Traditional Chinese medicine calls diabetes *Xiao ke zheng,* which includes diabetes insipidus — a disease characterized by the passage of large amounts of urine, and diabetes mellitus — a disease characterized by the presence of excessive amounts of sugar in the urine. Diabetes is a common disease of the internal system. It is manifested by various metabolic disorders and is caused by an insulin deficiency or by faulty utilization of insulin.

Patients of diabetes are often seen to lose weight, eat and drink enormously and urinate excessively. Besides, they often feel tired, have a numb feeling in the limbs, ache in the waist and back, etc. Man patients are often seen with impotence, and women with amenorrhoea.

The treatment of diabetes can usually be divided into dietetic treatment and medical treatment.

11.5.1 Dietetic treatment

Patients are advised to take a fixed amount of food at a fixed time of the day for each meal. They should eat more fruit, vegetables, and other high-protein food, and try to avoid high fat, high sugar, and high carbonhydrate food.

As dietetic treatment, patients may take the following food as suggested here.

Bitter gourd — Bitter gourds contain a kind of material which is similar to insulin and can help reduce blood sugar. Patients may take 60g of bitter gourds at every meal as a dish (three times a day). Bitter gourds may also be dried and made into powder. Patients may take 10g of the powder each time, three times a day.

Onion — The volatile oil in onions has the function of reducing blood sugar. Patients may eat 0.25 kg of stir-fried onions at each meal. Do not stew them.

Celery — Celery is among vegetables which contain the least carbonhydrate. Squeeze out the juice from 0.5 kg of fresh, raw celery. Take half of the juice in the morning, and the other half in the evening.

Finless eel — Finless eels contain an ingredient which can adjust sugar in the blood.

Chinese yam (*shan yao*) — Eat it steamed or boiled. Patients may have 50g of yam each time, three times a day. Another way to take it is to have equal amount of *Shan yao* and *Tian hua fen*, simmer them in water and then take 10g of the decoction each time, twice a day.

Beef — Beef is nourishing and produces no sugar in the urine. It's good food for patients of diabetes, but should be eaten with little soy sauce.

11.5.2 Medical treatment of diabetes

11.5.2.1 Example case 1
A man patient aged 50 had the following symptoms:
> drank enormously, urinated excessively, getting thinner and tired, felt hot in the chest, etc.

Prescription:
 Lü dou yi 12g   Sheng di huang 9g   Shi hu 9g
 Tian hua fen 12g   Huang lian 6g   Huang qin 9g
 Wu wei zi 6g   Mai dong 9g   Yuan shen 12g
 Shan yao 60g   Huang qi 30g   Dang shen 9g
 Shu di huang 9g

After taking eight dosages of the medicine, the patient felt better. Examination showed that albumen in the urine turned from ++++ to +, and blood sugar also decreased. But he still lacked appetite, felt thirsty and hot in the chest.

Second prescription:
 Sheng di huang 24g   Shu di huang 24g   Huang qi 60g
 Shou wu 12g   Bai zhu 12g   Shi gao 24g
 Ji nei jin 9g   Zhi mu 6g   Wu wei zi 9g
 Ren shen 6g   Mai dong 9g

The patient was recovered after taking ten dosages of the second prescription.

11.5.2.2 Example case 2

A man aged 29 was suffering from diabetes. He was getting thinner, and often felt tired and weak.

Prescription:
 Shan yao 60g   Huang qi 30g   Lü dou yi 12g
 Bai guo (14 pieces, beaten with shells)
 Nan hua fen 15g   Gou ji 15g   Dang shen 18g
 Shi hu 12g   Du zhong 9g   Xu duan 9g
 Shan zhu yu 12g
    (ten dosages)

Second prescription:
 Huang qi 30g   Shan yao 30g   Shan zhu yu 12g
 Dang shen 12g   Gua lou 9g   Tian hua fen 9g
 Du zhong 9g   Xu duan 9g   Ji li 9g

Sha ji li 9g   Shi hu 18g   Sheng di huang 6g
Shu di huang 6g   Sha ren 4.5g   Dang shen 12g
E jiao 9g   Sang ji sheng 24g   Bu gu zhi 9g
   (ten dosages)

Third prescription:
   Dang shen 12g   Huang qi 60g   Shan yao 30g
   Mai dong 9g   Tian dong 9g   Lü dou yi 12g
   Tian hua fen 15g   Shan zhu yu 15g   Wu wei zi 6g
   Shi hu 15g   Sheng di huang 15g   Ji li 9g
   Sha ji li 9g   Lu jiao jiao 9g
      (ten dosages)

The patient was fully recovered after taking the medicine.

11.5.2.3 Explanation of the main drugs used in the above prescriptions

Huang qi has the function of replenishing the vital energy and reducing blood sugar.

Huang qin is used to eliminate heat in the lung.

Huang lian is used to eliminate heat in the heart for insomnia, fidget, etc.

Lü dou yi is good to the spleen and stomach and can eliminate heat for the treatment of polydypsia.

Du zhong, Xu·duan and *Gou ji* are used to replenish the liver and kidney, to strengthen the bones and muscles for the treatment of aching back and knees.

Lu jiao jiao is a blood tonic.

Shi gao is used as antipyretic for heat in the lung and stomach with high fever, fidget and thirst.

Sheng di huang and *Shi hu* are used to nourish the vital essence for the treatment of its deficiency, to clear up the excessive heat and to promote the secretion of body fluids for the treatment of febrile diseases with thirst and dry mouth.

Bu gu zhi is used to warm up the kidney and to reinforce the vital function of the sexual organs for the treatment of impotence, etc.

11.6 TREATMENT OF UROLOGICAL DISEASES

Recorded here are five cases of five different kinds of urological diseases: hypertrophy of the prostate, renal calculus, orchitis, tubercular cystitis, and acute pyelitis.

11.6.1 A case of hypertrophy of the prostate
Name of patient: Gong   Age: 66   Sex: male
Symptoms: often had the desire to urinate but had very little urine; sometimes catheterization had to be used; had suffered from hypertrophy of the prostate for years.
The patient preferred taking herbal medicine to an operation.
Normal tongue coating, soft pulse.

Prescription:
   Che qian cao 9g   Han lian cao 9g   Fu ling 9g
   Chi xiao dou 18g   Hai fu shi 9g   Hai jin sha 9g
   Zhi mu 6g   Huang bai 6g   Wu zhu yu 6g
   Huang lian 6g   Hua shi 24g   Yu zhen gu 24g
   Sheng ma 3g   Gui zhi 5g   Wu yao 6g
   Gan cao 3g   Xi shuai 7g
      (two dosages)

The patient no longer had difficulty in urination after taking the medicine, but he still urinated frequently.

Second prescription:
   Sheng ma 3g   Gui zhi 5g   Chuan lian zi 6g
   Hai fu shi 6g   Hai jin sha 6g   Che qian cao 9g
   Han lian cao 9g   Yu zhen gu 24g   Hua shi 24g
   Fu ling 9g   Chi xiao dou 18g   Dong gua zi 12g
   Dong kui zi 12g   Wu zhu yu 5g   Huang lian 5g

Wu yao 6g   Gan cao 3g   Zhi mu 6g
Huang bai 6g   Lou gu 1g   Xi shuai 7g
(to be taken every other day, for thirty days or more)

Explanation note:
The prescriptions lay emphasis on solving difficulty in urination and urination disturbance such as pains during urination, dripping of urine, etc.

Sheng ma and *Gui zhi* are used to reolsve damp turbidity by invigorating vital function.

Diuretics are used, such as *Hai fu shi, Hai jin sha, Yu zhen gu, Hua shi, Fu ling, Ci xiao dou,* etc. They are for the treatment of acute infection of urinary system and caliculi of the urinary tract.

Zhi mu and *Huang bai* are antipyretics, used to eliminate heat and dampness for infection of the urinary system.

Wu zhu yu is used to relieve pain for the treatment of abdominal pain.

Lou gu and *Xi shuai* are used for retention of urine or renal failure with extreme suppression of urine secretion.

After taking the decoction for some time, the patient was recovered.

11.6.2   A case of renal calculus

A man named Liu, aged 40, had had an operation during which a kidney stone as big as a broad bean was taken out.

Recently he found blood in his urine, the amount of urine decreased and he had pain in the waist. The X-ray showed there were two renal calculuses in the ureter. His tongue coating was thin, white and slimy; his pulse soft and slippery. Sleep and diet normal.

Prescription:
Che qian cao 9g   Che qian zi 9g   Hai fu shi 9g
Hai jin sha 6g   Hua shi 18g   Wa leng zi 18g
Fu ling 12g   Jin qian cao 30g   Han lian cao 30g

E jiao 9g   Zhu ling 9g   Di yu 12g
Gou qi zi 9g   Dan cong rong 15g   Ze xie 9g
Gan cao 3g
   (seven dosages)

After taking the medicine, some sand-like things were passed out with urine. The X-ray showed there was still one calculus in the ureter but had moved down a bit.

Second prescription:
   Mang xiao 30g   Han lian cao 60g   Hua shi 60g
   Su mu 60g   Wa leng zi 30g   Hai fu shi 30g
   Zhu ling 30g   Ze xie 30g   Gou qi zi 60g
   Shan zhu yu 30g   E jiao 60g   Fu ling 30g
   Dan cong rong 60g   Tu si zi 60g   Zi cao 30g
   Di yu 60g   Qu mai 30g   Hai jin sha 30g
   Xu duan 30g   Du zhong 30g   Che qian zi 30g
   Gan cao 30g
      (To be powdered and mixed, and then be made into small pills after being mixed with 600g of *Jin ying zi gao*.
      Take 6g of the pills each time, once in the morning, once in the evening.)

The patient was also advised to drink daily as tea the water with 120g of *Jin qian cao* in it.

After the patient took the pills for 80 days, X-ray examination showed that the calculus had become even smaller and had moved further down in the ureter. But he still had pain in the lower abdomen and waist, and there was still blood in his urine when he had physical exercises.

Third prescription:
   Rou gui 30g   Mang xiao 60g   Zhi mu 30g
   Han lian cao 60g   Wa leng zi 30g   Chen xiang 15g
   Qing pi 15g   Dan cong rong 60g   Hua shi 60g
   Bi cheng qie 15g   Hai jin sha 30g   E jiao 60g
   Ze xie 30g   Tan xiang 15g   Mo yao 30g

Fu ling 60g   Hai fu shi 30g   Shan zhu yu 30g
Zi cao 30g   Tu si zi 60g   Yu zhen gu 30g
Wu yao 30g   Gan cao 30g

(Use honey as excipient and make the well-powdered and mixed drugs into "honeyed bolus", each weighing 9g.

Take one bolus each time, once in the morning once in the evening.)

Traditional Chinese medical classics had records of cases of renal calculus, and called such disease *Shi lin* — urinary disturbance associated with the presence of urinary calculi. Our present time has seen many cases of successful treatment of renal calculus with traditional Chinese medicine. However, further research needs to be done to find out why Chinese herbal medicine can turn calculi into "sand" which can be passed out with urine from the ureter.

11.6.3   A case of orchitis

Name of patient: Li   Age: 30   Sex: male
Symptoms: had suffered from orchitis for years; his testis was once injured and it was often swollen and straining because of cold and dampness; his pulse was deep and slow.

Prescription:
Ju he 9g   Li zhi he 9g   Xiao hui xiang 9g
Shan zha 30g   Ba ji tian 9g   Hu lu ba 6g
Fu zi 6g   Bai shao 9g   Hai fu shi 9g
Gui zhi 5g   Wa leng zi 30g   Sha ji li 9g
Ji li 9g   Shu di huang 9g   Sheng ma 3g
Jiu cai zi 6g   Chuan lian zi 9g   Gan cao 3g
Xi xin 3g
   (seven dosages)

Second prescription:
Ju he 6g   Li zhi he 6g   Bai shao 9g
Chai hu 3g   Xiao hui xiang 6g   Sha ji li 9g

Ji li 9g   Ba ji tian 9g   Hu lu ba 9g
Fu zi 9g   Dang gui 6g   Sheng ma 3g
Chuan lian zi 6g   Gan cao 3g
Rou gui 1.5g   Chen xiang 1.2g
  (These last two drugs should be powdered and divided into two equal amounts, ready to be used.
  When the got decoction of other drugs is ready, pour it over one share of the powder, stir the decoction, and then take it.)
     (seven dosages)

Third prescription:
  In the morning, take 9g of *Hui xiang ju he wan;* in the afternoon, take 6g of *Bu zhong yi qi wan;* before bed-time, take one pill of *Shen rong wei sheng wan* for 30 days.

Fourth prescription:
  In the morning, take 9g of *Hui xiang ju he wan;* in the afternoon, take 9g of *Jin gui shen qi wan;* before bed-time, take one pill of *Ren shen lu rong wan,* for 30 days.

Fifth prescription:
  Take medicine according to the fourth prescription for 30 more days.

The patient was fully recovered after that.
Traditional Chinese medicine calls testis the outer kidney, and believes that it is closely connected with the kidney.
When treating orchitis, drugs which can warm and tonify the vital function of the kidney are used.
Li's orchitis was first caused by external injury, and then by cold and dampness. As the disease lasted for a long time, pills (not decoction) were used. Though pills are usually slow in action, they are good at treating chronic diseases.

11.6.4   Treatment of tubercular cystitis
Name of patient: Peng   Age: 33   Sex: male

Symptoms: urination as frequent as 40 times a day, pain in the lower abdomen and ureter; sometimes had a chilly feeling in the back; urination with blood and turbid discharge, etc.

Peng had suffered from the disease for four years and felt it getting worse yearly.

Prescription:
   Che qian zi 9g   Che qiao cao 9g   Bi xie 9g
   Shi wei 9g   Sha ji li 9g   Ji li 9g
   Tong cao 9g   Bai shao 9g   Gui zhi 5g
   Sheng di huang 6g   Shu di huang 6g   Sha ren 5g
   Ju he 6g   Li zhi he 6g   Ban xia 9g
   Han lian cao 30g   Sheng qu 9g   E jiao 9g
   Gan cao 6g
      (four dosages)

Second prescription:
   Bai shao 9g   Gui zhi 3g   Chai hu 3g
   Du zhong 9g   Xu duan 9g   Sha ji li 9g
   Ji li 9g   Che qian cao 9g   Han lian cao 9g
   Bi xie 9g   She wei 9g   Ju he 6g
   Li zhi he 6g   Qing pi 5g   Guang pi tan 5g
   E jiao 9g   Sheng di huang 6g   Shu di huang 6g
   Sha ren 5g   Ba ji tian 6g   Ji nei jin 9g
   Fu zi 5g   Bai zhu 6g   Yi zhi ren 5g
   Gan cao 3g
      (six dosages)

After taking the medicine, the patient felt much better: there was no more turbid discharge with urine, and the pain stopped. He wanted to take pills to reinforce the effect.

Third prescription:
   In the morning, take one pill of *Bi xie fen qing wan,* in the evening before bed-time, take one pill of *Jin gui sheng qi wan,* for 30 days.

Explanation note:

Nephritis can be divided into acute and chronic cases. Acute nephritis is usually caused by external factors, while chronic nephritis is turned from acute nephritis or caused by pathological changes of the kidney. In treating nephritis, the doctor must first differentiate the cold, or heat, the deficiency or excessiveness symptom-complex. Cold symptom-complex should be treated with *Ma huang, Gui zhi, Fu zi, Xi xin,* etc. Heat symptom-complex should be treated with *Zhi mu, Huang bai, Huang qin, Huang lian, Shi gao,* etc. Deficiency symptom-complex should be treated with reinforcing or replenishing drugs, such as *Ren shen, Bai zhu, Huang qi,* etc. Excessiveness symptom-complex should be treated with *Zhu ling, Ze xie, Shang lu, Bian xu,* etc. To reinforce the vital function, we can use drugs like *Bu gu zhi, Ba ji tian, Rou gui,* etc. To replenish the vital essence, we can use drugs like *Shan zhu yu, Gou qi zi, Tu si zi, Shu di huang, Wu wei zi,* etc.

11.6.5 A case of acute pyelitis

Name of patient: Wang   Age: 30   Sex: female

Symptoms: frequent urination with turbid discharge, pain in the waist;

Laboratory test showed it to be acute pyelitis.

Prescription:

Che qian cao 9g   Han lian cao 9g   Yi yuan san 12g
Hai jin sha 9g   Xue yu tan 9g   Jiu cai zi 9g
Jin yin hua 12g   Bai mao gen 30g   Huang qin 6g
Huang bai 5g   Yi yi ren 12g   Ze xie 9g
Dan zhu ye 6g   Gan cao 3g   Fu ling 18g
Hu po 3g   (Powder *Hu po* first, divide it into two equal shares; then dissolve one share of the powder in the hot decoction of other drugs before taking.)

(four dosages)

Second prescription:
   Bi xie 9g   Shi wei 9g   Xue yu tan 9g
   Jiu cai zi 9g   Hai jin sha 9g   Hua shi 9g
   Jin yin hua 12g   Ze xie 9g   Wu yao 6g
   Yi yi ren 12g   Yi zhi ren 5g   Chang pu 5g
   Dan zhu ye 6g   Fu ling 9g   Mu tong 5g
   Bai mao gen 30g   Huang bai 5g   Gan cao 3g
      (four dosages)

Third prescription:
   In the morning, take *Bi xie fen qing wan* (one pill), in the evening, take one pill of *Zhi bai di huang wan,* for 10 days.

The patient was recovered after taking the medicine. According to Traditional Chinese medicine, in treating pyelitis, diuretic, antipyretic and antiphlogistic drugs should be used. *Jiu cai zi* can cure frequency of urine, when used with *Xue yu tan* it can treat inflammation of ureter. Big amount of *Bai mao gen* is effective in diminishing inflammation and stopping bleeding.
Xue yu tan is used as hemostatic and to eliminate blood stasis for the treatment of all kinds of bleeding.
Che qian cao and *Han lian cao,* when used together, can eliminate evil heat from the blood and tonify the kidney.
Hai jin sha is used to eliminate damp-heat and as lithagogue for the treatment of acute infections of urinary system and relieve pain.

11.7   TREATMENT OF IMPOTENCE

There are many things which may cause impotence. For instance, asthenia of the brain nerves may lead to asthenia of sex nerves. Impotence may also be caused by excessive fatigue, or heat and dampness, or anxiety and horror, etc. Deficiency of blood of the internal organs may also lead to impotence.

Impotence is often accompanied with the following symptoms: thin and cold seminal fluid, pain in the limbs, the back and waist, poor appetite, weariness, fidgety, etc.

11.7.1 Example case 1
The man patient, 48 years old, said to the doctor that he had been impotent for a year; his testes were icily cold, swollen and hurting sometimes; his heartbeat was 90 times per minute; he also suffered from amnesia, fidgety, dizziness, palpitation, varices and prospernia.

Prescription:
  Xian ling pi 60g   Xian mao 60g   Lu rong 30g
  Xiao hui xiang 30g   Ren shen 30g   Ju he 60g
  Hai ma 30g   Chuan lian zi 30g   Ji li 60g
  Gui zhi 30g   Fu zi 30g   Bai wei 30g
  Bu gu zhi 30g   Wu wei zi 30g   Yuan zhi 30g
  Sha ren 15g   Long gu 60g   Shan zhu yu 60g
  Shu di huang 60g   Rou gui 15g   Mu li 60g
  Fu ling 60g   Fu pen zi 30g   Jiu cai zi 30g
  Gan cao 30g   Ba ji tian 30g   Tu si zi 60g
  (To be powdered and well mixed, then made into pills each weighing 9g, with honey as excipient.
  Take one pill each time, once in the morning, once in the evening.)
  Note: these pills are enough to last the patient two months.

11.7.2 Example case 2
A Mr Hu, aged 56, had suffered from neurasthenia for years, and now was impotent. Whenever he got nervous, he would sweat. He had a bad appetite and indigestion.

Prescription:
  Xian ling pi 60g   Lu rong 60g   Ren shen 30g
  Ji li 60g   Xian mao 30g   Bai wei 30g

Gui zhi 30g   Bu gu zhi 60g   Jiu cai zi 30g
   Bai zhu 60g   Huang qi 60g   Dang gui 30g
   Fu pen zi 30g Wu wei zi 30g   Sha ren 15g
   Guang pi 15g   Di long 30g   Tu si zi 60g
   Yuan zhi 30g   Fu shen 60g   Shu di huang 30g
   Ba ji tian 60g Gan cao 30g

   (To be powdered and well mixed, and then made into pills, using as excipient the paste of 750g of *Shan yao*. Take 9g of the pills each time, once in the morning, once in the evening.)

After taking the medicine for two months, the patient felt much better: he could sleep five to six hours a day, had a better appetite and his ability to perform the sexual act was also improved.

Second prescription:
   Xi xian cao 60g   Zhi shi 60g   Lu rong 30g
   Xian ling pi 60g   Ren shen 30g   Xian mao 60g
   Ji li 60g   Gui zhi 30g   Bu gu zhi 60g
   Bai wei 30g Jiu cai zi 30g Bai zhu 60g
   Fu pen zi 30g Huang qi 60g Tu si zi 60g
   Bai shao 60g Fu shen 60g   Sha ren 15g
   Ba ji tian 60g Yuan zhi 30g Wu wei zi 30g
   Hai ma 15g   Shu di huang 30g Suan zao ren 60g
   Shan yao 90g   Gan cao 30g

   (To be powdered and well mixed, then made into pills each weighing 9g, using honey as excipient.
   Take one pill each time, twice a day.)

After taking the pills, which lasted him about 70 days, the patient was fully recovered.

11.8　TREATMENT OF DIARRHEA OF OLD PEOPLE

Name of patient: Xu　　Age: 63　　Sex: female
Symptoms: Had acute gastroenteritis, which turned into a

chronic case; passing loose, watery stools seven to eight times a day; cold in the stomach and abdomen; stuffed feeling in the chest; restless in sleep, etc.

Prescription:
   Ren shen 12g Wu wei zi 3g Fu zi 15g
   Mai dong 6g Yuan zhi 9g Gan cao 6g
   Gui zhi 6g
     (two dosages)

Second prescription:
   Fu zi 18g Wu wei zi 5g Fu ling 12g
   Gui zhi 9g Bai shao 9g Dang shen 15g
   Gan jiang 9g Bai zhu 9g Gan cao 6g
   Huang qi 24g Jie geng 5g Da zao 10(pieces)
     (two dosages)

Third prescription:
   Fu zi 30g Gan jiang 9g Da zao 10(pieces)
   Dang shen 30g Bai zhu 15g Gan cao 9g
     (two dosages)

Fourth prescription:
   Huang qi 30g Dang shen 30g Bai zhu 15g
   Dang gui 9g Gan cao 6g Wu wei zi 6g
     (two dosages)

Fifth prescription:
   Huang qi 60g Dang gui 30g Sheng jiang 30g
    Stew 180g of sliced mutton in water. When the soup is ready, take out the mutton slices and use the soup to simmer the drugs.
    Divide the decoction in two, take half in the morning, the other half in the evening.
      (two dosages)

Sixth prescription:
   Huang qi 60g   Dang shen 60g   E jiao 12g
   Lu jiao jiao 9g   Bai zhu 6g   Wu wei zi 3g
   Gan cao 9g   Da zao 10(pieces)
    (three dosages)

The patient was gradually improving after taking the medicine. Pain in the stomach stopped; her appetite was normal again; she passed stools, though still sticky loose sometimes, two to three times a day. Above all, she regained confidence in getting cured.

Seventh prescription:
   Huang qi 60g   Dang shen 60g   E jiao 12g
   Lu jiao jiao 9g   Mi qiao 9g   Wu wei zi 3g
   Gan cao 9g   Da zao 10(pieces)
    (three dosages)

The patient was fully recovered after taking the medicine.

Explanatory note:
   The patient was over 60 years old, and weak in body resistance. She was cold and deficient in the stomach and spleen, which was marked by chronic diarrhea, etc.
So, in all the prescriptions, drugs were used to warm and tonify the kidney, invigorate the function of the spleen, regulate the functioning of the spleen and stomach, and to reinforce the function of the heart. Thus the patient was finally cured.

11.9   TREATMENT OF OTITIS MEDIA

Name of patient: Jiang Lin   Age: 34   Sex: male
Symtoms: There was pus coming out from the right ear; and a numb and hot feeling in the ear; had been hard of hearing for a week; swelling in the ear had caused the patient hot and itching all over

and made him unable to sleep; etc.

Prescription:

Long dan cao 5g   Chan tui yi 5g   Bai wei 6g
Shi chang pu 6g   Da huang 6g   Ji li 12g
Niu xi 9g   Jie geng 5g   Lian qiao 9g
Ju hua 9g   Sang ye 9g   Cang er zi 6g
(two dosages)

After taking the medicine, the patient felt better: there was less pus from the ear, the hot and numb feeling was reduced, and he was better in hearing. However, itching rash appeared all over, and the skin felt hot.

Second prescription:

Pu gong ying 15g   Jie sui 6g   Cang er zi 6g
Lou lu 6g   Fu ling 6g   Chi shao 6g
Bai mao gen 12g   Sheng di huang 12g   Zi cao 6g
Zi hua di ding 6g   Fang feng 5g   Shi chang pu 6g
Chan tui yi 5g   Lian qiao 9g   Jie geng 5g
Jin yin hua 6g   Jin yin teng 6g   Shan zhi 6g
Gan cao 6g
(four dosages)

The medicine was effective: no more pus, most of the rash disappeared, hearing normal again. But itchiness remained; there was still some rash on his waist and lower limbs.

Third prescription:

In the morning, take 30 (small) pills of *Pi fu bing xue du wan,* in the afternoon, take 0.6g of *Qi bao miao ling dan,* before bed-time, take 30 (small) pills of *Pi fu bing xue du wan,* for 20 days.

Explanatory note:

To treat otitis media, the doctor should first ascertain the causes and symptoms of the disease and then give treatment. In the present case, mainly febrifugal and detoxicant drugs were used to remove toxic heat, diminish inflammation, dispel pathogenic wind to arrest itching and reduce swelling.

Pu gong ying and diminish inflammation and remove toxic heat.

Bai mao gen and *Sheng di huang*, when used together, can eliminate pathological heat from the blood so as to bring down the temperature.

Jie sui, Cang er zi, and *Fang feng can* dispel dampness and stop itching.

Jin yin hua and *Jin yin teng* can eliminate toxic heat (which causes inflammation), and clear up evil heat in channels and collaterals to kill the pain.

Shi cang pu and *Long dan cao* can help clear the channels in the ear.

Lao zong tan and *Niu xi* are used to lead evil heat downward to diminish inflammation in the ear.

The patient was basically cured after taking six dosages of the decoction. Almost all the symptoms of otitis disappeared, only some rash remained. Pills, which were taken for 20 days, reinforced the effect of the decoction and cured the remaining rash.

11.10 TREATMENT OF GOUT

Gout is usually caused by cold and dampness, which penetrate into the body when the patient's body resistance is weak (such as when living in a cold and damp place for a long time, or catching cold in a storm.) This may lead to disorder of metabolism. Its main symptoms are: intensely painfulness and swelling in the joints, red and swollen and feeling hot in some parts of the body, etc.

11.10.1 Example case 1
Name of patient: Chu   Age: 30   Sex: female
Symptoms: painful in the upper limbs; the right arm ached so much that it could not be lifted, etc.

Prescription:
 Bai shao 9g   Gui zhi 3g   Di long 9g
 Sheng di huang 9g   Shu di huang 9g   Xi xin 1.5g
 Chuan xiong 5g   Du huo 5g   Dang gui 9g
 Xuan fu hua 6g   Yiu song jie 15g   Hong hua 6g
 Jiang huang 6g   Shen jin cao 9g   Qian nian jian 9g
 Gan cao 6g

The patient took two dosages of the medicine first, and felt better. So she took ten more dosages according to the prescription and was recovered after that.

11.10.2 Example case 2
Name of patient: Liu Zhicai   Sex: male
Symptoms: joints had been aching for months, felt most painful in the waist and hipbone, etc.
Prescription:
 Sang zhi 18g   Sang ji sheng 18g   Du zhong 6g
 Xu duan 6g   Bai shao 9g   Gui zhi 3g
 Sheng di huang 6g   Shu di huang 6g   Xi xin 3g
 Sha ren 3g   Chuan xiong 5g   Di long 9g
 Yiu song jie 30g   Du huo 5g   Mu gua 9g
 Dang gui 9g   Gou ji 15g   Gong lao ye 12g
 Qin jiao 5g   Che qian cao 9g   Han lian cao 9g
 Gan cao 10g
  (three dosages)

After taking the medicine, some itching rash appeared, and the pain in the knee-joints and right hand seemed to be worse than before. But the pain in other parts was relieved.

Second prescription:
 Bai shao 6g   Shen di huang 9g   Shu di huang 9g
 Ji li 9g   Sha ji li 9g   Sang ye 6g
 Sang ji sheng 18g   Hei zhi ma 24g   Jin jie sui 6g
 Chuan xiong 5g   Du huo 5g   Gou ji 5g
 Che qian cao 9g   Han lian cao 9g   Dang gui 9g

Yiu song jie 30g   Gu ya 9g   Mai ya 9g
Gan cao 10g
   (three dosages)

Itching rash disappeared after taking the medicine, and pain in the joints was reduced. Only the right knee ached more. The patient slept better and had a better appetite.

Third prescription:
Ju hong 5g   Ju luo 5g   Xuan fu hua 6g
Zhe shi 9g   Sang ye 6g   Sang ji sheng 18g
Hei zhi ma 24g   Gou ji 15g   Gong lao ye 12g
Sha ren 5g   Dou kou 5g   Wei ling xian 6g
Yiu song jie 30g   Sha ji li 9g   Ji li 9g
Dang gui 6g   Di long 9g   Gan cao 10g
Bai shao 9g   Gui zhi 5g   Yuan zhi 9g
   (three dosages)

The patient felt much better after taking the medicine, but wanted to take some pills to reinforce the effect.

Fourth prescription:
Hei zhi ma 30g   Sang ye 30g   Gou ji 30g
Hu gu 30g   Di long 30g   Sheng di huang 30g
Shu di huang 30g   Sha ji li 30g   Du huo 15g
Qin jiao 15g   Bai shao 30g   Chai hu 15g
Du zhong 30g   Dang gui 30g   Chuan xiong 15g
Lu jiao jiao 15g   Sha ren 15g   Yuan zhi 30g
Gan cao 30g
   (To be powdered and mixed and then made into pills, each weighing 9g, with the paste of 360g of *Shan yao* as excipient.
   Take one pill every morning and evening.)

11.10.3 Explanation of the property and action of the drugs in treating gout

Du huo and *Qin jiao* are used as antirheumatic and

analgesic agents for the treatment of rheumatic pain.

Gui zhi, Xi xin, and *Fang feng* are used to warm and clear out the channels and rheumatic arthritis.

Chi shao, Dang gui, Hong hua and *Chuan xiong* can invigorate blood circulation, and so are used to remove stagnated blood and eliminate evil heat from the blood for the treatment of pains due to blood-stasis.

Huang qi, Dang shen, Bai zhu can invigorate the functions of the spleen and stomach, so are used to treat symptoms due to deficiency of vital energy of these viscera (such as poor appetite, loose bowels, etc.) They can also help increase body resistance.

Shu di huang and *Xi xin* are used to replenish the vital essence of the kidney, to nourish the blood, and fill the marrow for the treatment of pain of the waist.

In the first stage of the disease, emphasis should be laid on dispelling the invading pathogenic factors. But in chronic cases, emphasis should be laid on strengthening the patient's resistance. Only when the doctor makes the correct diagnosis of the disease, can he choose the right therapeutic method. (See Chapters 5 and 6.)

11.11 TREATMENT OF DYSMENORRHOEA

Dysmenorrhoea is caused when the flow of blood and vital energy is blocked or impeded. Patients are often seen to have intense pain during menstruation, a painful and stuffed feeling in the sides, nausea, etc.

In treating dysmenorrhoea, drugs should be used mainly to invigorate blood circulation, regulate the flow of vital energy, warm up the spleen and stomach and to dispel the internal cold.

11.11.1   Example case 1

Name of patient: Miss Li   Age: 23
Symptoms: had suffered from dysmenorrhoea for years; had pain in the lower abdomen before each menstruation; the blood was dark purple with lumps in it, etc.
colour of tongue: dark purple
tongue coating: thin and white
pulse: deep and thin (as fine as a silk thread)

Prescription:
  Yi mu cao 12g Yuan hu 6g Ai ye 5g
  Dang gui 9g Sheng di huang 6g Shu di huang 6g
  Bai shao 12g Chuan xiong 5g Shan zhu yu 12g
  Sha ren 5g Chai hu 5g Qing pi 5g
  Bu gu zhi 6g E jiao 9g Gan cao 3g
  Sheng jiang 1g Da zao 5 (pieces)
    (three dosages)

This medicine should be taken five days before menstruation each month, for three successive months.

For patients who prefer taking patent pills, the following pills are recommended.

In the morning, take one pill of *Ai fu nuan gong wan;* in the evening, take one pill of *Fu ke de sheng dan.*

The patient should also start taking medicine five days before menstruation each month. She should take the pills for ten days running each time, for three successive months. In most cases, the patient would be recovered after taking the medicine.

11.11.2 Example case 2

Name of patient: Miss Feng   Age: 18
Symptoms: had suffered from dysmenorrhoea, which caused such pain that she couldn't work as usual.

Prescription:
  Dan shen 30g Dang gui 12g Hong hua 9g
  Tao ren 9g Xiang fu 9g Ze lan 9g
  Wu yao 9g Gan cao 3g Qing pi tan 6g

Chen pi tan 6g   Ai ye 5g   Bai shao 9g
Chai hu 5g
(the medicine is taken the same way as in Example case 1)

Explanatory note:

Dan shen, Dang gui, Ze lan, Tao ren, Hong hua can invigorate blood circulation and eliminate blood-stasis. *Dang gui* is the most effective and most important drug in treating women diseases as it can nourish the blood, invigorate the functioning of the heart, help get rid of blood-stasis and produce new blood.

Qing pi, Chen pi, Wu yao can regulate the flow of vital energy for the treatment of abdominal pain.

Bai shao and *Chai hu* can nourish and tonify blood. They can also coordinate the exterior and interior.

There are also some pain-killers used: *Xiang fu* (invigorate blood circulation and kill pain), *Wu yao, Ai ye* (warm the lower abdomen, dispel cold and kill pain), *Dang gui, Yi mu cao* (can regulate the menstrual flow for the treatment of abnormal menstruation), and *Yuan hu* (relieve all kinds of pain with a sedative effect.)

11.12   TREATMENT OF TUBERCULAR ERYTHEMA

Name of patient: Miss Wang Yiren   Age: 24
Symptoms: retarded menstruation, dark coloured blood; legs and feet had been swollen for half a month with purple erythema, the skin on which had come off; poor appetite; pain in the waist and back; cough, nausea, etc.
Prescription:
Sang ye 6g   Sang ji sheng 18g   Qian hu 5g
Bai qian 5g   Zi yuan 5g   Hua hong 5g
Hou po hua 5g   Mei gui hua 5g   Bai shao 6g

Gui zhi 5g   Sha ji li 9g   Ji li 9g
Jie geng 5g   Qin jiao 5g   Dang gui 6g
Lu gen 9g   Sheng di 9g   Dai dai hua 6g
Yue ji hua 6g   Jin jie sui 6g   Chai hu 5g
Gan cao 3g   Tao ren 6g   Xing ren 6g
  (four dosages)

After taking the medicine, the swelling came down; the colour of the spots turned from purple to red. But she still had a stuffed feeling in the chest, and her waist and back still ached.

Second prescription:
Cang zhu 6g   Bai zhu 6g   Sang ye 6g
Sang ji sheng 18g   Sha ji li 9g   Ji li 9g
Chi shao 6g   Bai shao 6g   Gui zhi 0.6g
Hou po hua 5g   Mei gui hua 5g   Jin jie sui 6g
Dang gui 6g   Chuan xiong 5g   Hou po 5g
Tao ren 6g   Xing ren 6g   Gou ji 15g
Sheng di huang 9g   Di long 9g   Gan cao 3g
Shan zha 9g   Chai hu 5g
  (three dosages)

Some red spots disappeared, but some remained. At night, legs and feet swelled a little bit. She also had a headache and some pain in the chest.

Third prescription:
Ji li 30g   Sha ji li 30g   Long chi 30g
Dang gui 30g   Dang shen 30g   Dan shen 30g
Gou ji 30g   Sheng di huang 30g   Shu di huang 30g
Chi shao 30g   Bai shao 30g   Chuan xiong 15g
Sha ren 15g   Jin jie sui 30g   Zi he che 30g
Lu jiao jiao 30g   E jiao 30g   Hong hua 15g
Bai zhu 30g   Ai ye 15g   Yuan hu 30g
Yi mu cao 60g   Gan cao 15g   Mu gua 30g
Fang ji 30g   Huang qi 60g

(To be powdered and mixed, and then made into pills with honey as excipient.
Take 9g of the pills each time, every morning and evening.)

The pills lasted the patient about one and half months. After taking the medicine, she was recovered.

11.13 TREATMENT OF PURPURA

Purpura means the occurrence of multiple small purplish haemorrhages in the skin and mucous membranes, due to a variety of blood and blood vessel disorders.

The following is the record of the treatment of a case of a plastic anaemia.

Name of patient: Liu Ruiming   Age: 11   Sex: male
Main information and symptoms of the disease:

He was hospitalized last spring for nasal bleeding. The blood examination at the outpatient department this time (1955) showed his haemochrome was under 3g, time of haemorrhage was 8.5 minutes, and time of coagulation was 3.5 minutes. Purpura appeared on his gums and purple blisters on his tongue. He was often dizzy and tired. The pulse on his right wrist was full and the pulse on the left was fine, which showed deficiency of vital energy and blood. He was taken in hospital.

Prescription:
Xian he cao 15g   Pu huang 6g   Da ji 6g
Xiao ji 6g   Long gu 12g   Mu li 12g
Zi cao 9g   Han lian cao 9g   Bai wei 5g
Zi yuan 5g   Fu ling 6g   Chi shao 6g
Sheng ma 3g   Jin jie sui 3g   Gan cao 3g
Dan pi 6g   Huang qi 15g   E jiao 6g
Chai hu 3g

(Lu jiao jiao 3g. Gui ban jiao 3g. These drugs should be simmered separately but taken with the decoction of the other drugs.)

After taking two dosages of the medicine, the patient felt better. There was no more bleeding at day time.

Second prescription:
    Long gu 12g   Mu li 12g   Sheng di huang 6g
    Shu di huang 6g   Sheng ma 3g   Sha ren 3g
    Bai qian 5g   Zi yuan 5g   E jiao 6g
    Pu huang 9g   Wu bei zi 5g   Wu wei zi 3g
    Chi shao 9g   Bai shao 9g   Chai hu 5g
    Zi hua di ding 9g   Zi cao 6g   Ge gen 6g
    Shan zhi 3g   Da ji 6g   Xiao ji 6g
    Ce bai ye 6g   Jiao san xian 9g   He ye 9g
    Chi shi zhi 9g

(When the decoction is ready, add in the separately simmered or steamed
    Lu jiao jiao 4.5g   Gui ban jiao 4.5g
before taking.)
    (three dosages)

Bleeding was still not stopped totally after taking the medicine. To stop bleeding, drugs should be used first to regulate the functioning of the five viscera and warm the channels.

Third prescription:
    Dai ge san 9g   Tie luo 9g   Sheng ma 3g
    Jin jie sui 3g   Bai qian 5g   Zi yuan 5g
    Zhu ma gen 6g   Niu xi 5g   Ku xing ren 5g
    Sheng di huang 12g   Bai mao gen 12g   Pu gong ying 9g
    Pu huang 9g   Sang ji sheng 15g   Sang piao xiao 5g
    Xian he cao 12g   Zi cao 6g   Sang bai pi 5g
    Chun gen pi 5g   Dan pi 6g   Gan cao 3g
    Da ji 6g   Xiao ji 6g   Sha shen 6g

Yuan shen 6g   E jiao 6g   Ma bo 5g
(two dosages)

Fourth prescription:
Hua rui shi 5g   Zhu ma gen 5g   Shi gao 15g
Xue yu tan 3g   Tie luo 9g   Xian he cao 9g
Han lian cao 9g   Zi cao 6g   Zi yuan 6g
Ou jie tan 15g   Fang feng 3g   Ku xing ren 5g
Sang bai pi 5g   Sang ji sheng 18g   Qian hu 5g
Bai qian 5g   Zhi mu 5g   Bei mu 5g
Lu jiao jiao 6g   E jiao 6g   Huang qi 15g
Sheng jiang 3g   Zhu ye 5g   Zhu ru 5g
Huang qin 6g   Chi shi zhi 9g   Xiao ji 6g
(three dosages)
(Before taking the decoction each time, take 0.8g of powdered *San qi* which should be put in capsules with warm boiled water.)

The medicine was effective. After taking the medicine, most of the purpura was assimilated.

Fifth prescription:
Lu jiao jiao 6g   E jiao 6g   Ce bai tan 6g
He ye tan 6g   Bai qian 5g   Zi yuan 5g
Fu ling 6g   Chi shao 6g   Sheng ma 3g
Jin jie sui 3g   Sha shen 5g   Yuan shen 5g
Long gu 9g   Mu li 9g   Sang bai pi 5g
Dan pi 5g   Gan cao 3g   Zi cao 6g
Wu wei zi 3g   Ge gen tan 6g   Ci zhu wan 9g
Xue yu tan 5g   Chi shi zhi 6g   Hua rui shi 6g
(three dosages)

After taking the medicine, bleeding and coughing stopped. Stools were sticky loose and blackish yellow.

Sixth prescription:
Xue yu tan 5g   Chen cang mi 6g   Long gu 9g

Mu li 9g　Di jin cao 6g　Xian he cao 9g
Bai jiang cao 9g　Ju hua 9g　Jin yin hua 9g
Shu di huang 9g　Sha ren 3g　Ce bai tan 6g
Di yu tan 6g　Ge gen tan 5g　Sheng ma 5g
Lian xu 6g　Huang qi 15g　Lu jiao shuang 5g
E jiao 6g　Zi cao 5g　Zi yuan 5g
Xin yi 3g　Xiao ji 6g　Chi shi zhi 6g
　(five dosages)

The patient regained his appetite after taking the medicine. His stools returned to normal.

Seventh prescription:
　E jiao 6g　Lu jiao jiao 3g　Gui ban jiao 3g
　　(These three drugs should be simmered or steamed separately and then taken with the decoction of the other drugs.)
　Long yan rou 9g　Di jin cao 9g　Huang qi 15g
　Dang gui 6g　Xian he cao 9g　Hua rui shi 9g
　Dang shen 9g　Long gu 9g　Mu li 9g
　Wu bei zi 3g　Wu wei zi 3g　Bai shao 9g
　Chai hu 3g　Zi hua di ding 9g　Dan shen 9g
　Sheng di huang 6g　Chuan xiong 3g　Zi yuan 5g
　Bai wei 5g　Sheng ma 3g　Jin jie sui 3g
　Zi cao 6g　Gan cao 3g
　　(five dosages)

The patient felt well again after taking the medicine and rested for two days without taking any medicine. But he still wanted to take some more decoctions to reinforce the effect.

Eighth prescription:
　Long gu 9g　Mu li 9g　Gui ban 9g
　Bie jia 9g　Sheng di huang 5g　Shu di huang 5g
　Xi xin 1.5g　Sheng ma 3g　Chi shi zhi 9g
　Hua rui shi 9g　Shan zhu yu 9g　Fu ling 6g
　Chi shao 6g　Cang er zi 5g　Tu si zi 5g

Ce bai tan 6g   Pu huang 6g   Zi yuan 5g
Zi cao 5g   Yuan shen 6g   Niu xi 5g
Huang qi 18g   Dang gui 6g   Di gu pi 5g
Shan yao 18g   Dan pi 5g   Gan cao 3g
   (five dosages)

The patient was practically well again and so was discharged from hospital. He was advised to go on taking:
   in the morning, *Ren shen yang rong wan* 6g,
   in the evening, *Quan lu wan* 5g,
   for 20 days.
The whole course of treatment lasted about a month.

11.14 TREATMENT OF TYPHUS

Name of patient: Mr Cao
Symptoms: had suffered from influenza with stomach trouble; had high fever for a week, obstruction of stool, hiccup, thick, slimy tongue-coating, pain in the joints, etc.
Prescription:
   Lu gen 12g   Bai mao gen 12g   Xuan fu hua 6g
   Zhe shi 6g   Can sha 9g   Zao jiao zi 9g
   Huang qin 9g   Huang lian 5g   Gua lou 24g
   Xie bai 9g   Dan dou chi 9g   Zhi qiao 5g
   Jie geng 5g   Ku xing ren 6g   Pei lan 9g
   Yu jin 9g   Shi di 9g   Shan zhi 6g
   Ji nei jin 9g   Gan cao 3g
      (two dosages)

Evil heat was not cleared up: there were some red spots on the skin, tongue-coating was still thick, stools were dry and hard, urine was reddish brown, etc.

Second prescription:
   Sheng di huang 12g   Zi hua di ding 6g   Zi cao 6g
   Lu gen 12g   Bai mao gen 12g   Can sha 9g

Zao jiao zi 9g   Fu ling 9g   Chi shao 9g
Shan zhi 6g   Jin jie sui 6g   Pei lan 9g
Dan pi 9g   Sang ye 6g   Sang zhi 18g
Zhi qiao 5g   Chan tui yi 5g   Lian qiao 9g
Gan cao 3g
  (two dosages)
  (Each time with the decoction, take 1.5g of *Zi xue san* as extra conductant ingredient.)

The dry and hardened stool was discharged, but the patient still had a high fever.

Third prescription:
  Two more dosages of medicine according to the second prescription.

The fever gradually came down. But bowels movement was not yet free. Mr Cao was hard of hearing and sometimes made delirious speech.

Fourth prescription:
  Shan zhi 6g   Dan dou chi 9g   Pei lan 9g
  Lu gen 12g   Bai mao gen 12g   Sheng di huang 12g
  Fu ling 9g   Chi shao 6g   Huang qin 6g
  Huang lian 3g   Jin jie sui 6g   Ku xing ren 6g
  Dan pi 6g   Jie geng 5g   Chan tui yi 5g
  Chang pu 5g   Gan cao 3g
    (two dosages)

Fifth prescription:
  Shi hu 12g   Sheng di huang 12g   Fu ling 9g
  Mai dong 9g   Chang pu 6g   Gu ya 9g
  Mai ya 9g   Ji li 9g   Lü e mei 9g
  Yuan zhi 9g   Suan zao ren 12g   Hou po hua 6g
  Mei gui hua 6g   Bai shao 9g   Nuo dao gen 12g
  Gan cao 3g   Sha shen 12g
    (four dosages)

Mr Cao was recovered after taking the medicine.

Appendix

English and/or Latin Names of Chinese Drugs in Common Use

A

Ai fu nuan gong wan 艾附暖宮丸
　Pills for women's diseases with argyi, etc.

　Ingredients:
　　Ai ye, Xiang fu, Huang qi, Rou gui, Dang gui, Yuan hu, Wu zhu yu, etc.

Ai ye 艾葉
　Argyi Leaf; Chinese Mugwort Leaf
　Folium Artemisiae Argyi

B

Ba ji tian 巴戟天
　Morinda Root
　Radix Morindae Officinalis

Bai bian dou 白扁豆
　White Hyacinth Bean
　See also *Bian dou*

Bai dou kou ren, Bai kou ren, Bai dou kou 白荳蔻仁，白蔻仁，白荳蔻
　Round Cardamom Seed
　Semen Cardamomi Rotundi

Bai fan 白矾
　Alum
　Alumen

Bai guo 白菓
　Ginkgo Seed
　Semen Ginkgo

Bai he 百合
　Lily Bulb
　Bulbus Lilii

Bai ji 白及
　Bletilla Tuber
　Rhizoma Bletillae

Bai ji li 白蒺藜
　See also *Ji li*

Bai jiang can, Jiang Can 白僵蠶，僵蠶
　Batryticated Silkworm, White-stiff Silkworm
　Bombyx Batryticatus

Bai Jiang Cao 敗醬草
　Patrinia Herb
　Herba Patriniae

Bai kou ren 白蔻仁
　See also *Bai dou kou ren*

117

Bai li 白梨
　Pear Syrup

Bai mao gen 白茅根
　Imperata Rhizome; Cogongrass Rhizome
　Rhizoma Imperatae

Bai qian 白前
　a perennial mountain grass, the root of which is used as antitussive and expectorant, and a diuretic
　Rhizoma Cynanchi Stauntonii

Bai shao 白芍
　White Peony Root
　Radix Paeoniae Alba

Bai wei 白薇
　Swallowwort Root
　Radix Cynanchi Atrati

Bai zhi 白芷
　Dahurian Angelica Root
　Radix Angelicae Dahuricae

Bai zhu 白朮
　White Atractylodes Rhizome
　Rhizoma Atractylodis Macrocephalae

Bai zi ren 柏子仁
　Arborvitae Seed
　Semen Biotae

Ban lan gen 板藍根
　Isatis Root, Dyer's Woad Root
　Radix Isatidis

Ban xia 半夏
　Pinellia Tuber
　Rhizoma Pinelliae

Bao he wan 保和丸
　Pills for keeping the functioning of the stomach in good condition
　Ingredients:
　　Shan zha, Shen qu, Lai fu zi, Fu ling, Chen pi, Ban xia, Lian qiao

Bei chi 貝齒
　See also *Zibei chi*

Bei mu 貝母
　See also *Chuan bei mu*, and *Zhe bei mu*

Bei sha shen, Sha shen 北沙參
　Glehnia Root
　Radix Glehniae

Bi bo 蓽茇
　Long Pepper
　Fructus Piperis Longi

Bi chen qie 畢澄茄
　Litsea cubeba fruit
　Fructus Litseae

Bi xie 萆薢
　There are two kinds of *Bie xie* with the same function:
　Mian bi xie, Seven-lobed Yam; Rhizoma Dioscoreae Septemlobae
　Fen bi xie, Hypoglauca Yam; Rhizoma Dioscoreae Hypoglaucae

Bi xie fen qing wan 萆薢分清丸
　Pills for eliminating infections of the urinary system with Dioscorea septemloba, etc.

　Ingredients:
　　Bi xie, Yi zhi ren, Shi chang pu, Wu yao, etc.

Bian dou, Bai bian dou 扁豆，白扁豆
　Hyacinth Bean, Lentil
　Dolichos Lablab

Bian dou yi 扁豆衣
　the shell of the beans

Bian dou hua 扁豆花
　the white flowers of the bean

Bian xu 扁蓄
  Common Knot-grass
  Herba Polygoni Avicularis

Bie jia 鱉甲
  Turtle Shell
  Carapax Trionycis

Bing lang 檳榔
  Betal nut; Areca Seed
  Semen Arecae

Bo he 薄荷
  Peppermint
  Herba Menthae

Bu gu zhi 補骨脂
  Psoralea Fruit
  Fructus Psoraleae

Bu xin dan 補心丹
  Mind-easing Tonic Pills

  Ingredients:
    Fu ling, Ren shen, Mai dong, Suan zao ren, Bai zi ren, Yuan zhi, Dang gui, etc.

C

Can sha 蠶砂
  Wilkworm Excrement
  Excrementum Bombycis

Can tui, Can yi, Can tui yi
  蟬蛻，蟬衣，蟬蛻衣
  Cicada Slough; Cicada Skin
  Periostracum Cicadae

Cang er zi 蒼耳子
  Xanthium Fruit; Cocklebur Fruit
  Fructus Xanthii

Cang pu 菖蒲
  See also *Shi cang pu*

Cang zhu 蒼朮
  Atractylodes Rhizome
  Rhizoma Atractylodis

Cao dou kou 草豆蔻
  Katsumadai Seed
  Semen Alpiniae Katsumadai

Cao jue ming 草決明
  Cassia Seed
  Semen Cassiae

Cao wu 草烏
  Wild Aconite Root
  Radix Aconiti Kusnezoffii

Ce bai ye 側柏葉
  Biota Tops; Arborvitae Tops
  Cacumen Biotae

Cha ye 茶葉
  Tea leaves

Chai hu 柴胡
  Bupleurum Root; Thorowax Root
  Radix Bupleuri

Che qian cao 車前草
  Plantain Herb
  Herba Plantaginis

Che qian zi 車前子
  Plantain Seed
  Semen Plantaginis

Chen cang mi 陳倉末
  Limonite
  Limonitum

Chen pi 陳皮
  Tangerine Peel
  Pericarpium Citri Reticulatae

Chen xiang 沉香
  Eagle Wood
  Lignum Aquilariae Resinatum

Chi shao 赤芍

Red Peony Root
Radix Paeoniae Rubra

Chi shi zhi 赤石脂
Red Halloysite
Halloysitum Rubrum

Chi xiao dou 赤小豆
Phaseolus Seeds; Adsuki Bean
Semen Phaseoli

Chong wei zi 茺蔚子
the seeds of *Yimucao*
Motherwort Seeds
Fructus Leonuri

Chuan bei mu, Bei mu 川貝母，貝母
Tendrilled Fritillary Bulb
Bulbus Fritillariae Cirrhosae

Chuan lian zi 川楝子
Sichuan Chinaberry
Fructus Meliae Toosendan

Chuan mu tong 川木通
See also *Mu tong*

Chuan niu xi 川牛膝
Cyathula Root
Radix Cyathulae

Chuan po 川樸
See also *Hou po*

Chuan shan jia 穿山甲
Pangolin Scales
Squama Manitis

Chuan wu 川烏
Sichuan Aconite Root
Radix Aconiti

Chuan xiong 川芎
Chuanxiong Rhizome
Rhizoma Liguistici Chuanxiong

Chun bai pi, Chun gen pi 椿白皮，椿根皮
Ailanthus Bark, Tree of Heaven Bark
Cortex Ailanthi

Ci gu cao 茨菇草
Spodiopogon Sagittifolius Rendle

Ci shi 磁石
Magnetite
Magnetitum
(a kind of magnetic iron ore Fe_3O_4)

Ci wei pi 刺猬皮
dried Hedgehog Skin
Corium Erinacei

Ci zhu wan 磁硃丸
Sedative Pills of Magnetitum and Cinnabaris

Ingredients:
Ci Shi, Zhu sha, Sheng qu

D

Da huang 大黃
Rhubarb
Radix et Rhizoma Rhei

Da ji 大薊
Japanese Thistle
Herba seu Radix Cirsii Japonici

Da zao 大棗
Jujube; Chinese Date
Fructus Ziziphi Jujubae

Dai dai hua 玳玳花
a kind of fragrant yellowish white flowers grown in Zhejiang (Chekiang) province, etc.

Dai zhe shi 代赭石
See also *Zhe shi*

Dan dou chi 淡豆豉
 Prepared soybean
 Semen Sojae Praeparatum

Dan pi, Mu dan pi 丹皮，牡丹皮
 Moutan Bark; Tree Peony Bark
 Cortex Moutan Radicis

Dan shen 丹參
 Red Sage Root
 Radix Salviae Miltiorrhizae

Dan zhu ye 淡竹葉
 Lophatherum
 Herba Lophatheri

Dang gui 當歸
 Chinese Angelica Root
 Radix Angelicae Sinensis

Dang shen 黨參
 Pilose Asiabell Root
 Radix Codonopsis Pilosulae

Dao ya 稻芽
 Germinated Rice
 Fructus Oryzae Germinatus

Di fu zi 地腹子
 Broom Cypress Fruit
 Furctus Kochiae

Di gu pi 地骨皮
 Wolfberry Bark
 Cortex Lycii Radicis

Di jin cao 地錦草
 See also *Wo dan cao*

Di long 地龍
 Earth-worm
 Lumbricus

Di yu 地榆
 Sanguisorba Root; Burnet Root
 Radix Sanguisorbae

Ding xiang 丁香
 Cloves
 Flos Caryophylli

Dong gua zi 冬瓜子
 Seed of Chinese Waxgourd
 Semen Benincasae

Dong kui zi 冬葵子
 Seed of Sunflower

Du huo 獨活
 Pubescent Angelica Root
 Radix Angelicae Pubescentis

Du zhong 杜仲
 Eucommia Bark
 Cortex Eucommiae

Duan mu li, Mu li 斷牡礪，牡礪
 Ignited Oyster Shell
 Concha Ostreae Usta

E

E jiao, Lu pi jiao 阿膠，驢皮膠
 Donkey-hide Gelatin; Ass-hide Glue
 Colla Corii Asini

E zhu 莪朮
 Zedoary
 Rhizoma Zedoariae

Er chou 二丑
 See also *Qian niu zi*

F

Fang feng 防風
 Ledebouriella Root
 Radix Ledebouriellae

Fang ji 防己
 Tetrandra Root
 Radix Stephaniae Tetrandrae

121

Feng huang yi 鳳凰衣
Egg's lining membrane

Feng xian hua zi 風箱花子
See also *Jixing zi*

Fu ling, Fu shen 茯苓，茯神
Tuckahoe
Poria

Fu pen zi 覆盆子
Raspberry Fruit
Fructus Rubi

Fu ping 浮萍
See also *Zi fu ping*

Fu shen 茯神
See also *Fu ling*

Fu shou 佛手
Finger Citron
Fructus Citri Sarcodactylis

Fu xiao mai 浮小麥
Light Wheat
Fructus Triciti Levis

Fu zi 附子
Prepared Aconite Root
Radix Aconiti Praeparata

G

Gan cao 甘草
Liquorice; Licorice Root
Radix Glycyrrhizae

Gan jiang 乾薑
Dried Ginger
Rhizoma Zingiberis

Gan song 甘松
Nardostachys Rhizome; Spikenard Rhizome
Rhizoma Nardostachyos

Gao ben 藁本
Ligusticum Root
Rhizoma et Radix Ligustici

Gao liang jiang 高良薑
Rhizome Lesser Galangal
Rhizoma Alpiniae Officinari

Ge gen 葛根
Pueraria Root
Radix Puerariae

Ge gen tan 葛根炭
Charred (carbonized) Pueraria Root

Gong lao ye 功勞葉
the leaves of a kind of ever green arbor grown in Jiangsu province, China, used as antirheumatics

Gou ji, Jin mao ji 狗脊，金毛脊
Cibot Rhizome
Rhizoma Cibotii

Gou qi zi 枸杞子
Wolfberry Fruit
Fructus Lycii

Gou teng 鈎藤
Uncaria Stem with Hooks
Ramulus Uncariae cum Uncis

Gu ya 谷芽
Germinated Millet
Fructus Setariae Germinatus

Gua lou 瓜蔞
Trichosanthes Fruit; Snakegourd Fruit
Fructus Trichosanthis

Gua lou gen 瓜蔞根
See also *Tian hua fen*

Guang ji sheng 廣寄生
See also *Sang ji sheng*

Guang mu xiang 廣木香
  Costusroot
  Saussurea Lappa

Guang pi 廣皮
  See also *Chen pi*

Gui ban 龜板
  Tortoise Plastron; Terrapin Shell
  Plastrum Testudinis

Gui ban jiao 龜板膠
  Gelatinated Tortoise Plastrum, Tortoise Plestron Glue

Gui zhi 桂枝
  Cinammom Twigs; Cassia Twigs
  Ramulus Cinnamomi

H

Hai fu shi 海浮石
  Coral (stonelike substance formed from the bomes of very small sea animals – Polyps)

Hai jin sha 海金沙
  Lygodium japonicum; Japanese Fern Spores
  Spora Lygodii

Hai ma 海馬
  Sea-horse
  Hippocampus

Hai piao xiao 海螵蛸
  Cuttlefish Bone
  Os Sepiellae seu Sepiae

Hai zao 海藻
  Seaweed
  Sargassum

Han lian cao 旱蓮草
  Eclipta
  Herb Ecliptae

He shou wu 何首烏
  See also *Shou wu*

He tao ren 核桃仁
  Persian Walnut; Seed of English Walnut
  Semen Juglandis

He ye 荷葉
  Lotus Leaf
  Folium Nelumbinis

He ye tan 荷葉炭
  Charred Lotus Leaf

He zi 訶子
  Chebula Fruit
  Fructus Chebulae

Hei dou 黑豆
  Black Soya Bean

Hei zhi ma 黑芝蔴
  Black Sesame Seeds

Hong hua, Zang hong hua 紅花，藏紅花
  Safflower
  Flos Carthami

Hong qi 紅七
  Hedysarum Root
  Radix Hedysari

Hong ren shen 紅人參
  A kind of Genseng, which is steamed when raw and then dried

Hou po, Chuan po 厚樸，川樸
  Magnolia Flowers (dried)
  Cortex Magnoliae Officinalis

Hu gu 虎骨
  Tiger's Bone

Hu lu ba 胡蘆巴
  Fenugreek Seed
  Semen Trigonellae

Hu po 琥珀
  Amber
  Succinum

Hua rui shi 花蕊石
  Ophicalcite
  Ophicalcitum

Hua shi 滑石
  Talc
  Talcum

Huai niu xi 准牛膝
  See also *Niu xi*

Huang bai 黄柏
  Phellodendron Bark
  Cortex Phellodendri

Huang jing 黄精
  Siberian Solomonseal Rhizome
  Rhizoma Polygonati

Huang lian 黄蓮
  Coptis Root
  Rhizoma Coptidis

Huang qi 黄芪
  Astragalus Root
  Radix Astragali seu Hedysari

Huang qin 黄芩
  Scutellaria Root; Baikal Skullcap Root
  Radix Scutellariae

Huang yuan hua 黄芫花
  Chamaedaphne Leaf and Flower; Yellow Genkwa Leaf and flower
  Folium et Flos Wikstroemiae Chamaedaphnis

Hui xiang ju he wan 茴香菊核丸
  Pills for treating pain of testicles and hernia
  Ingredients:
  Xiao hui xiang, Ju he, Yuan hu, Kun bu, Li zhi he, Chuan lian zi, Mu xiang, etc.

Huo xiang 藿香
  Agastache; Wrinkled Giant hyssop
  Herba Agastachis

J

Ji cai 薺菜
  Capsella; Shepherd's Purse
  Herba Capsellae

Ji li, Bai ji li 蒺藜，白蒺藜
  Tribulus Fruit; Puncturevine Fruit
  Fructus Tribuli

Ji nei jin 鷄内金
  Chicken's Gizzard-skin
  Endothelium Corrneum Gigeriae Galli

Ji xing zi, Feng xian hua zi 急性子，風箱花子
  Garden Balsam Seeds
  Semen Impatientis

Ji xue teng 鷄血籐
  Spatholobus Stem
  Caulis Spatholobi

Jian qu 箭麯
  See also *Shen qu*

Jiang can 僵蠶
  See also *Bai jiang can*

Jiang huang 羌黄
  Turmeric
  Rhizoma Curcumae Longae

Jiang xiang 降香
  Dalbergia Wood
  Lignum Dalbergiae Odoriferae

Jiang zhong po 薑仲樸
   Hou po soaked and preserved in ginger and then dried

Jiao san xian 焦三仙
   Charred Triplet (a mixture consisting charred medicated leven, crataegus fruit and germinated barley)

Jie geng 桔梗
   Platycodon Root; Balloonflower Root
   Radix Platycodi

Jie sui 芥穗
   See also *Jing jie sui*

Jin deng long 錦燈籠
   Winter Cherry Fruit
   Calyx seu Fructus Physalis

Jin gui shen qi wan (also called *Fu gui ba wei wan*) 金匱腎氣丸
   Pills for restoring vital energy and function of the kidney
   Ingredients:
      Fu zi, Rou gui, Shu di huang, Wu zhu yu, Shan yao, Fu ling, Mu dan pi.

Jin mao ji 金毛脊
   See also *Gou ji*

Jin qian cao 金錢草
   Lysimachia
   Herba Lysimachiae

Jin yin hua 金銀花
   Honeysuckle flower
   Flos Lonicerae

Jin yin teng 金銀藤
   Honeysuckle stem
   Caulis Lonicerae

Jin ying zi 金櫻子
   Cherokee Rose-hip
   Fructus Rosae Laevigatae

Jing da ji 金大戟
   Peking Spurge Root
   Radix Euphobriae Pekinensis

Jing jie 荊芥
   Schizonepeta
   Herba Schizonepetae

Jing jie sui 荊芥穗
   Spike of Schizonepeta

Jiu cai zi 韭菜籽
   Chinese chives seeds

Ju he 橘核
   Tangerine Seed
   Semen citri Reticulatae

Ju hong 橘紅
   Pummelo Peel
   Exocarpium Citri Grandis

Ju hua 菊花
   Chrysanthemum Flower
   Flos Chrysanthemi

K

Ku fan 苦矾
   Calcined Alum (calcined *Bai fan*)

Ku shen 苦參
   Flavescent Sophora Root
   Radix Sophorae Flavescentis

Ku ding cha 苦丁茶
   Ilex cornuta
   Lindl

Ku xing ren, Xing ren 苦杏仁，杏仁
   Bitter Apricot Kernel
   Semen Armeniacae Amarum

Kun bu 昆布
　　Laminaria; Ecklonia
　　Thailus Laminariae seu Eckloniae

L

Lai fu ying 萊服英
　　Radish Leaf (dried leaves of garden radish)
　　Folium Raphani

Lai fu zi 萊服子
　　Radish Seed
　　Semen Raphani

Lao zong tan 老棕炭
　　Carbonized Petiole of Windmill-palm
　　Petiolus Trachycarpi Carbonisatus

Li zhi he 李子核
　　Litchi Seed; Lychee Seed
　　Semen Litchi

Lian qiao 連壳
　　Forsythia Fruit
　　Fructus Forsythiae

Lian xu 連鬚
　　Stamen Nelumbinis

Ling yang jiao 羚羊角
　　Antelope's Horn
　　Cornu Antelopis

Liu huang, Tian shen huang
琉璜，天生璜
　　Sulphur
　　Sulfur

Long chi 龍齒
　　Dragon's Teeth (the fossil teeth of ancient large mammals)
　　Dens Draconis

Long dan cao 龍胆草
　　Chinese Gentian
　　Radix Gentianae

Long gu 龍骨
　　Dragon's Bone (the fossil bone of ancient large mammal, such as Stegodon orientalis and Rhinocerus sinensis)
　　Os Draconis

Long yan rou 龍眼肉
　　Longan Aril
　　Arillus Longan

Lou gu 螻蛄
　　Mole Cricket
　　Gryllotalpa

Lou lu 漏蘆
　　A kind of wet grass grown in marshland, the root is used.

Lu gen 蘆根
　　Reed Rhizome
　　Rhizoma Phragmitis

Lu hui 蘆薈
　　Aloes (the dried leaf juice of Aloe)
　　Aloe

Lu jiao 鹿角
　　Antler; deerhorn
　　Cornus Cervi

Lu jiao jiao 鹿角膠
　　Antler Glue
　　Colla Cornus Cervi

Lu jiao shuang 鹿角霜
　　Deglued Antler Powder
　　Cornu Cervi Degelatinatum

Lu rong 鹿茸
　　Pilose Antler; Pilose Deerhorn
　　Cornu Cervi Pantotrichum

Lü dou 綠豆

Mung bean; Green gram

Lü dou yi 綠豆衣
　Skin of green gram or mung beans

Lü e mei 綠萼梅
　Mume Flower; Japanese Apricot Flower
　Flos Mume

Lü pi jiao 驢皮膠
　See also *E jiao*

M

Ma bian cao 馬鞭草
　Verbain
　Herba Verbenae

Ma bo 馬勃
　Puff-ball
　Lasiosphaera seu Calvatia

Ma huang 麻黃
　Ephedra
　Herba Ephedrae

Mai dong 麥冬
　Ophiopogon Root; Lilyturf Root
　Radix Ophiopogonis

Mai ya 麥芽
　Germinated Barley
　Fructus Hordei Germinatus

Man jing zi 蔓荊子
　Vitex Fruit
　Fractus Viticis

Mang xiao 芒硝
　Mirabilite; Sodium Sulphate
　Natrii Sulfas

Mei gui hua 玫瑰花
　Roses
　Rugosa Rose

Mi cu 米醋
　Rice Vinegar

Mi qiao 米壳
　Poppy Capsule
　Pericarpium Papaveris

Min jiang 闽薑
　Xian jiang macerated (or soaked) in sugar

Mo yao 沒藥
　Myrrh; Myrrha
　Resina Myrrhae

Mu dan pi 牡丹皮
　See also *Dan pi*

Mu gua 木瓜
　Chaenomeles Fruit; Flowering-quince Fruit
　Fructus Chaenomelis

Mu li 牡蠣
　Oyster Shell
　Concha Ostreae

Mu tong, Chuan mu tong 木通，川木通
　Clematis Stem
　Caulis Clematidis Armandii

Mu xiang 木香
　Aucklandia Root
　Radix Aucklandiae

N

Nan hua fen 南花粉
　See also *Tian hua fen*

Niu bang zi 牛蒡子
　Arctium Fruit; Burdock Fruit
　Fructus Arctii

Niu huang 牛黃
　Ox Gallstone

127

Calculus Bovis

Niu xi, Huai niu xi 牛膝，准牛膝
Achyranthes Root
Radix Achyranthis Bidentatae

Nü zhen zi 女貞子
Lucid Ligustrum Fruit; Grossy Privet Fruit
Fructus Ligustri Lucidi

Nuo dao gen 糯稻根
Glutinous rice root

O

Ou jie 藕節
Lotus Node
Nodus Nelumbinis Rhizomatis

P

Pei lan, Pei lan yi 佩蘭，佩蘭葉
Eupatorium
Herba Eupatorii

Pi fu bing xue du wan 皮膚病血毒丸
Pills for skin disease by removing toxic heat in the blood

Main ingredients:
Yi mu cao, Ji xue teng, Chan tui yi, Hong hua, Fu ling, Yin hua, Lian qiao, Di fu zi, etc.

Pi pa ye 枇杷葉
Loquat Leaf
Folium Eriobotryae

Po gong yin 蒲公英
Dandelion
Herba Taraxaci

Q

Qi bao miao ling dan 七寶妙齡丹
Pills for invigorating the functioning of the stomach

Ingredients:
Chen xiang, She xiang, Hou po, Fu ling, etc.

Qian cao, Qian cao gen 茜草，茜草根
Rubia Root; Madder Root
Radix Rubiae

Qian hu 前胡
Peucedanum Root; Hogfennel Root
Radix Peucedani

Qian nian jian 千年健
Homalomena Occulta Schott
Rhizoma Homalomenae

Qian niu zi, Er chou 牽牛子，二丑
Morning Glory Seeds
Semen Pharbitidis

Qian shi 芡實
Euryale Seed
Semen Euryales

Qiang huo 羌活
Notopterygium Root
Rhizoma seu Radix Notopterygii

Qin jiao 秦艽
Large-leaf Gentian Root
Radix Gentianae Macrophyllae

Qing pi 青皮
Green Tangerine Peel
Pericarpium Citri Reticulatae Viride

Qing pi tan 青皮炭
Carbonized Pangerine Peel

Qu mai 瞿麥
Pink (it consists of the dried aerial parts of Fringed Pink)
Herba Dianthi

Quan lu wan 全鹿丸
　Deer Tonic Pills

　Ingredients:
　　Ren shen, Lu rong, Suo yang, Ba ji tian, Dang gui, Chen xiang, Shu di huang, etc.

Quan xie 全蝎
　Scorpion
　Scorpio

R

Ren dong hua 忍冬花
　See also *Jin yin hua*

Ren dong teng 忍冬籐
　See also *Jin yin teng*

Ren shen 人參
　Ginseng
　Radix Ginseng

Ren shen lu rong wan 人參鹿茸丸
　Ginseng Antler Pills

　Ingredients:
　　Ren shen, Lu rong, Du zhong, Dang gui, Ba ji tian, Niu xi, Gui yuan rou, etc.

Rou cong rong 肉蓯蓉
　Cistanche Stem
　Herba Cistanchis

Rou dou kou, Rou guo 肉豆蔻，肉果
　Nutmeg
　Semen Myristicae

Rou gui 肉桂
　Cinnamon Bark; Cassia Bark
　Cortex Cinnamomi

Rou guo 肉果
　See also *Rou dou kou*

Ru xiang 乳香
　Frankincense
　Olibanum; Resina Olibani

S

San leng 三棱
　Burreed Tuber
　Rhizoma Sparganii

San qi 三七
　Notoginseng
　Radix Notoginseng

Sang bai pi 桑白皮
　Mulberry Bark
　Cortex Mori Radicis

Sang ji sheng 桑寄生
　Mulberry Mistletoe
　Ramulus Loranthi

Sang piao xiao 桑螵蛸
　Mantis Egg-case
　Oötheca Mantidis

Sang ye 桑葉
　Mulberry Leaf
　Folium Mori

Sang zhi 桑枝
　Mulberry Twig
　Morus Alba

Sha ji li, Sha yuan zi 沙蒺藜，沙苑子
　Flattened Milkvetch Seed
　Semen Astragali Complanati

Sha ren 砂仁
　Amomum Fruit
　Fructus Amomi

Sha shen 沙參
　See also *Bai sha shen*

Sha yuan zi 沙苑子

See also *Sha ji li*

Shan yao 山藥
　Chinese yam
　Rhizoma Dioscoreae

Shang yu rou 山萸肉
　See also *Shan zhu yu*

Shan zha 山楂
　Hawthorn Fruit
　Fructus Crataegi

Shan zhi 山梔
　Cape Jasmine Fruit
　Fructus Gardenia

Shan zhu yu, Shan yu rou
　山茱萸，山萸肉
　Dogwood Fruit
　Fructus Corni

Shang lu 商陸
　Phytolacca Root; Pokeberry Root
　Radix Phytolaccae

She xiang 麝香
　Musk
　Moschus

Shen jin cao 伸筋草
　Club-moss
　Herba Lycopodii

Shen jing shuai ruo wan 神經衰弱丸
　Anti-Neurasthenia Pills

　Ingredients:
　　Ci shi, Shu wu teng, Huang jing, Dan shen, Suan zao ren, Dang gui, Yuan wu wei zi, etc.

Shen qu 神麯
　Medicated Leaves
　Massa Fermentata Medicinalis

Sheng di, Sheng di huang 生地，生地黃
　Rehmannia Root
　Radix Rehmanniae

Sheng jiang 生薑
　Fresh Ginger
　Rhizoma Zingiberis Recens

Sheng ma 升麻
　Cimicifuga Rhizome
　Rhizoma Cimicifugae

Shen rong wei sheng wan 參茸衛生丸
　Ginseng and Pilose Antler Life-preserving Pills
　Ingredient:
　　Ren shen, Lu rong, Lian zi, Suan zao ren, Suo yang, Ba ji tian, Gou qi zi, etc.

Shi cang pu, Cang pu 石菖蒲，菖蒲
　Grass-leaved Sweetflag Rhizome
　Rhizoma Acori Graminei

Shi di 柿蒂
　Kaki Calyx; Persimmon Calyx
　Calyx Kaki

Shi gao 石膏
　Gypsum
　Gypsum Fibrosum

Shi hu 石斛
　Dendrobium
　Herba Dendrobii

Shi jue ming 石決明
　Sea-ear Shell
　Concha Haliotidis

Shi lian rou 石蓮肉
　Dried Seeds of Lotus

Shi wei 石韋
　Pyrrosia Leaf
　Folium Pyrrosiae

Shou wu, He shou wu 首烏，何首烏

Fleeceflower Root
Radix Polygoni Multiflori

Shou wu teng 首烏籐
Fleeceflower Stem
Caulis Polygoni Multiflori

Shu di, Shu di huang 熟地，熟地黃
Prepared Rehmannia Root
Radix Rehmanniae Praeparata

Shu mi 秫米
Husked Sorghum

Shuang gou teng 雙鉤籐
Ramulus Uncariae cum Uncis

Su he xiang 蘇合香
Styrax
Styraxi; Styrax Liquidus

Su mu 蘇木
Sappan Wood
Lignum Sappan

Su zi, Zi su zi 蘇紫，紫蘇紫
Perilla Seed
Fructus Perillae

Suan zao ren 酸棗仁
Wild (Spiny) Jujuba Seed
Semen Ziziphi Spinosae

Suo yang 鎖陽
Cynomorium
Herba Cynomorii

T

Tai zi shen 太子參
Pseudostellaria Root
Radix Pseudostellariae

Tan xiang 檀香
Sandal Wood
Lignum Santali Albi

Tao ren 桃仁
Peach Kernel; Peach Seed
Semen Persicae

Tian dong 天冬
Asparague Root
Radix Asparagi

Tian hua fen 天花粉
Trichosanthes Root; Snakegourd Root
Radix Trichosanthis

Tian ma 天麻
Gastrodia Tuber
Rhizoma Gastrodiae

Tian sheng huang 天生磺
See also *Liu huang*

Ting li zi 葶藶子
Lepidium Seed
Semen Lepidii seu Descurainiae

Tong cao 通草
Ricepaper Pith
Medulla Tetrapanacis

Tu fu ling 土茯苓
Smilax Glabra Rhizome
Rhizoma Smilacis Glabrae

Tu si zi 菟絲子
Dodder Seed
Semen Cuscutae

W

Wa leng zi 瓦楞子
Ark Shell
Concha Arcae

Wei ling xian 威靈仙
Clematis Root
Radix Clematidis

Wo dan cao, Di jin cao 卧胆草，地錦草
　Euphorbia Humifusa
　Herba Euphorbiae Humifusae

Wu bei zi 五倍子
　Chinese Nut-gall
　Galla Chinensis

Wu gong 蜈蚣
　Centipede
　Scolopendra

Wu ling zhi 五靈脂
　Trogopterus Dung
　Faeces Trogopterorum

Wu wei zi 五味子
　Schisandra Fruit; Magnoliavine Fruit
　Fructus Schisandrae

Wu yao 烏葯
　Lindera Root; Spicebush Root
　Radix Linderae

Wu zhu yu 吳茱萸
　Euodia Fruit
　Fructus Euodiae

X

Xi shuai 蟋蟀
　Dried Cricket

Xi xian cao 豨薟草
　Siegesbeckia Herb; St. Paulswort
　Herba Siegesbeckiae

Xi xin 細辛
　Asarum Herb; Wind Ginger
　Herba Asari

Xi yang shen 西洋參
　American Ginseng
　Radix Pancis Quinquefolii

Xia ku cao 夏枯草
　Prunella Spika; Selfheal Spike
　Spica Prunellae

Xian he cao. 仙鶴草
　Agrimony
　Herba Agrimoniae

Xian ling pi 仙靈脾
　Epimedium
　Herba Epimedii

Xian mao 仙茅
　Curculigo Rhizome
　Rhizoma Curculiginis

Xian ren tou 仙人頭
　The turnip after being blossomed and seeded

Xiang fu, Xiang fu tan 香附，香附炭
　Cyperus Tuber; Flatsedge Tuber
　Rhizoma Cyperi

Xiang ru 香薷
　A kind of fragrant grass; its stem is used to treat influenza
　Herba Elsholtziae seu Moslae

Xiang sha yang wei wan 香砂養胃丸
　Stomachic Pills with Cyperus and Amomam

　Ingredients:
　　Xiang fu, Sha ren, Mu xiang, Bai zhu, Chen pi, Hou po, etc.

Xiang yuan 香櫞
　Citron
　Fructus Citri

Xiao hui xiang 小茴香
　Fennel Fruit
　Fructus Poeniculi

Xiao ji 小薊
　Cephalanoplos Herb
　Herba Cephalanoploris

Xie bei 薤白
  Small Thistle
  Bulbus Allii Macrostemi

Xin yi 辛夷
  Magnolia Flower
  Flos Magnoliae

Xing ren 杏仁
  See also *Ku xing ren*

Xiong dan 熊胆
  Bear Gall
  Fel Ursi

Xu duan 續斷
  Dipsacus Root; Teasel Root
  Radix Dipsaci

Xuan fu hua 旋復花
  Inula Flower
  Flos Inulae

Xuan ming fen 玄明粉
  Dried Glauber's Salt; Exsiccated Sodium Sulfate
  Natrii Sulfas Exsiccatus

Xuan shen 玄參
  See also *Yuna shen*

Xue jie 雪竭
  Dragon's Blood
  Sanguis Draconis

Xue yu tan 雪餘炭
  Carbonized Hair
  Crinis Carbonisatus

Y

Yan hu suo 延胡素
  See also *Yuan hu*

Yi mu cao 益母草
  Motherwort
  Herba Leonuri

Yi yi ren 薏苡仁
  Coix Seed; Job's-tears Seed
  Semen Coicis

Yi yuan san 益元散
  Yi yuan powder *(Hua shi, Gan cao, Zhu sha)*

Yi zhi ren 益智仁
  A kind of fragrant grass; its seeds contain terpen and assquiterpen

Yin chen 茵陳
  Oriental Wormwood
  Herba Artemisiae Scopariae

You song jie 油松節
  node of pine tree

Yu jin 鬱金
  Curcuma Root
  Radix Curcumae

Yu zhen gu 魚枕骨
  the stone-like thing in the head of yellow croaker

Yu zhu 玉竹
  Fragrant Solomonseal Rhizome
  Rhizoma Polygonati Odorati

Yuan hu, Yan hu suo 元胡,元胡素
  Corydalis Tuber
  Rhizoma Corydalis

Yuan hua 芫花
  Genkwa Flower
  Flos Genkwa

Yuan ming fen 元明粉
  See also *Mang xiao, Xuan ming fen*

Yuan shen, Xuan shen 元參,玄參
  Scrophularia Root; Figwort Root
  Radix Crophulariae

Yuan zhi 遠志
   Polygala Root
   Radix Polygalae

Yue ji hua 月季花
   Chinese Rose
   Flos Rosae Chinensis

Z

Zang hong hua 藏紅花
   Saffron
   Stigma Croci; Crocus

Zao jiao ci 皂角刺
   Honeylocust Thorn
   Spina Gleditsiae

Zao jiao zi 皂角籽
   the seeds of Chinese Honeylocust

Ze lan 澤蘭
   Bugleweed
   Herba Lycopi

Ze xie 澤瀉
   Alisma Rhizome; Water-plantain Tuher
   Rhizoma Alismatis

Zhe bei mu 浙貝母
   Thunberg Fritillary Bulb
   Bulbus Fritillariae Thunbergii

Zhe shi, Dai zhe shi 赭石，代赭石
   Hematite
   Haematitum

Zhi bai di huang wan 知柏地黃丸
   Pills to nourish vital essence and diminish pathogenic fire with Anemarrhena Rhizome and Phellodendron Bark

   Ingredients:
      Zhi mu, Huang bai, Shu di huang, Shan zhu yu, Shan yao, Ze xie, Dan pi, Fu ling.

Zhi mu 知母
   Anemarrhena Rhizoma
   Rhizoma Anemarrhenae

Zhi qiao 枳壳
   Bitter Orange
   Fructus Aurantii

Zhi shi 枳實
   Immature fruit of Bitter Orange
   Fructus Aurantii Immaturus

Zhu ling 猪苓
   Umbellate Pore Fungus
   Polyporus Umbellatus

Zhu ma gen 苧蔴根
   Boemeria Root; Ramie Root
   Radix Boehmeriae

Zhu ru 竹茹
   Bamboo Shavings
   Caulis Bambusae in Taeniam

Zhu sha 朱砂
   Cinnabar
   Cinnabaris

Zhu sha an shen wan 朱砂安神丸
   Sedative pills with Cinnabar, etc.

   Ingredients:
      Zhu sha, Huang lian, Dang gui, Shu di huang, etc.

Zi bei chi, Bei chi 紫貝齒，貝齒
   Purple Cowrie; Purple Cowry Shells
   Concha Mauritiae

Zi cao 紫草
   Arnebia Root; Lithosperm Root
   Radix Arnebiae seu Lithospermi

Zi fu ping, Fu ping 紫浮萍，浮萍
   Duckweed

Zi he che 紫河車
   Dried Human Placenta
   Placenta Hominis

Zi hua di ding 紫花地丁
   Viola Herb; Yedoens Violet
   Herba Violae

Zi shi ying 紫石英
   Amethyst

Zi su ye 紫蘇葉
   Perilla Leaf
   Polium Perillae

Zi su geng 紫蘇根
   Perilla Stem

Zi su zi 紫蘇籽
   See also *Su zi*

Zi yuan 紫苑
   Aster Root
   Radix Asteris

Zi xue san 紫雪散
   Purple Snowy Powder for Clearing Evil Heat and Inducing Sedation

   Ingredients:
     Xi jiao, Ling yang jiao, She xiang, Chen xiang, etc.

Zuo jin wan 左金丸
   Pills for Clearing Up Evil Heat of the Liver and Invigorating the Functioning of the Stomach

   Ingredients:
     Huang lian, Wu zhu yu